THE
NEW PATIENT
AVALANCHE SYSTEM

CHIROPRACTIC MARKETING HANDBOOK

THE
NEW PATIENT
AVALANCHE SYSTEM

The Exact Marketing
Blueprint That Helped Me Scale
to 8 Practices and Over 11,000
New Patients Every Year

Dr Ryan Rieder

Praise For Ryan Rieder and The New Patient Avalanche Program (From Chiropractors <u>All Over The World</u>)

"Ryan's taking chiropractic marketing to an absolute business level. We've generated 87 NP and we haven't even finished the course yet!!!"

Dr Andrew Jackson

"Just counted our stats for Aug and Sept with NPA ... 213 leads from the stuff we learnt on the New Patient Avalanche Course and, of those, 79 New Patient bookings so far – WOW!"

Dr Brian and Ciara Mc Elroy

"Since we started coaching with Ryan, my clinic has exploded ... Over the last month we have had our busiest 4-week period EVER (New Patients and Adjustments) ... We are generating an EXTRA $7600 PER WEEK ... ($380 000+ per year increase)."

Dr Mike Paull

"One of the best, an inspiration to so many to impact more lives."

Dr Dan Knowles

"I've just recently finished Ryan's New Patient Avalanche Program and it's the best course HANDS DOWN I've ever done with regards to marketing. I used to think I was pretty good at marketing, but working with Ryan we've managed to get that extra 20-30%."

Dr Charles Herbert

"It was quite transformational for our practice (New Patient Avalanche) ... During one week of doing the course we added 30 New Patients ... We did a great internal promotion during the course and added another 20 New Patients to our practice ... We now have a Facebook ad that every time we switch it on, we get 15 New Clients JUST FROM THAT!"

Charlotte McCrossin

"We had an increase of 60 New Patients in 4 weeks!!! We can increase by a minimum of 720 new patients over the year just by implementing this stuff ... wow."

Dr Alex and Nick Smiljanic

"It's been one of the most influential courses I have taken in my life. Ryan really is THE REAL DEAL when it comes to marketing, to mindset and to growing your clinic."

Dr Jonny Coller

"I've been working with Ryan for 4 months and what I like about him is just his honesty and that he's ACTUALLY DOING IT, HE'S IN THE TRENCHES."

Paul Musk

THE MOST INCREDIBLE FREE GIFT EVER!

GET 3 MONTHS FREE MEMBERSHIP

Learn how to claim your $441 worth of pure, powerful, practice-growing material absolutely FREE! Get our monthly 25+ page "Practice Growth Playbook" sent straight to your door!

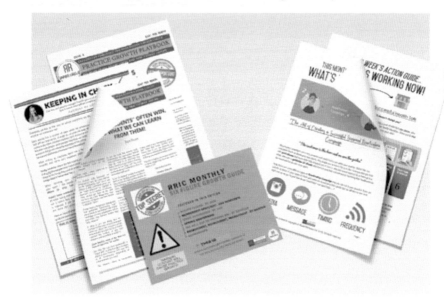

GO TO NPAMARKETINGBOOK.COM/PRACTICE-GROWTH-PLAYBOOK TO UNLOCK YOUR FREE BONUS OR EMAIL INFO@DCPRACTICEGROWTH.COM

CLAIM YOUR AMAZING FREE BONUS

Access your live bonus training of the Facebook platform

- ✓ Learn how to double your new patients using Facebook

- ✓ Learn how to get 60-100 new leads on Facebook in days

- ✓ See the benefits of using Facebook in your practice

- ✓ Spread your message to a whole new audience

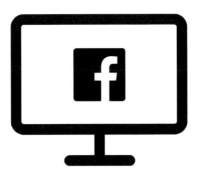

GO TO NPAMARKETINGBOOK.COM TO UNLOCK YOUR FREE BONUS OR EMAIL INFO@DCPRACTICEGROWTH.COM

CONTENTS

INTRODUCTION

As professionals, it's our duty to share the magic of chiropractic with as many people as possible.

We also want to do that in a way that helps us build a successful business that delivers the lifestyle we want for ourselves and our teams.

The key to achieving those objectives is a steady stream of the right kind of clients – or an avalanche as I prefer to call it.

In this book, I'm going to be sharing the exact strategies that have helped me build Halsa into one of the UK's prominent chiropractic businesses, with eight offices, 11,000 new clients every year and over 7 million dollars in revenue each year.

I'm going to show you exactly what we did so that you can use our experience and learning to build your practice.

But I'll say one important thing. If you're looking for that elusive silver bullet that is going to make growing your practice easy, you're looking in the wrong place because quite frankly it doesn't exist. Trust me I have looked.

The truth is, I promise you, you'll go through this book and, at some point, you will want to kick yourself, because you're going to go, "Oh my word. I do know that but I've stopped doing it for some reason."

One of my greatest teachers taught me that knowing and not doing is the same as not knowing. So, there's going to be things you read that make you go, "My word, I forgot about that," and that's perhaps going to be your biggest breakthrough.

The book is split into two segments:

1. **Marketing Fundamentals:** I've found that many people rush straight into implementing marketing tactics without taking time to build firm foundations.

2. **New Patient Avalanche Blueprint:** This is the exact marketing blueprint that I follow to regularly generate 11,000 new clients every single year.

My strategies are by no means the only way to generate new clients and referrals for your practise. There are many ways to skin a cat as they say, but these tried and tested bankers are things that have served me well.

These are tried and tested bankers that give you the biggest bang for your buck and helped me build a 1% business.

I promise you, that if you try doing every marketing campaign out there, it will be very overwhelming, and the key is to get the biggest bang for your buck, which you're going to learn in this book.

This helped me build a one percent business. What is a one percent business? There's only one percent of businesses on the planet that ever reach above $5 million turnover per annum and I'm going to teach you the exact strategies that helped us achieve this throughout the book.

PART ONE

THE FUNDAMENTALS OF MARKETING AND PREPARING YOUR NEW PATIENT AVALANCHE

PREPARING YOURSELF FOR THE NEW PATIENT AVALANCHE

One of my biggest frustrations coaching people about growing their chiropractic business is that they rush too quickly into doing things without having the proper fundamentals in place.

If you don't establish firm foundations, it's very difficult for us to set you up for a win.

So, before we go in to the details of what you need to do, I want to spend some time getting the fundamentals right.

One of the most important foundations of success is getting the right mindset and starting to like a business owner or strategist as appose to just a good operator.

Being Ready for the Challenge

When I was planning this book, I sent several people a questionnaire about their marketing challenges and business challenges and I'd like to share some of them with you.

I'm not going to go list them all, but it doesn't matter where you practice or what you specialise in, these are some of the common ones.

Marketing Challenges

- Finding time to do marketing
- Developing the 'How to' knowledge
- Maintaining consistency
- Having a clear message the public will understand
- Creating a sound marketing strategy

- Prioritizing what to do first
- Overcoming fears around promoting self and "sales talk"
- Calculating of how and what to spend money on
- Not knowing what to do, where to start
- Technical know-how

Business Challenges

- Running a team
- Wearing too many hats
- Clarity of vision
- Failure to think like a CEO and just focussing on short term
- Belief in self and the limits of my current personal development
- Planning and managing staff and building the culture
- Doing the work while finding time to work on the business
- Not having the finances available to invest in the business for the future
- Finding employees that have the drive to help build your business
- Building the business to a level that fills the diary weeks in advance

There are lots of different issues there, but I can honestly sum all of those into up with one word, OVERWHELM.

We get overwhelmed and what happens when we suffer overwhelm in business is we end up looking and acting like a deer in the headlights and we just don't do anything.

One of my aims in this book is to help you beat the overwhelm.

Some of the ways I'll do that are by helping you decide what's important and focus on that and also giving you a head start by helping you get clear what to do next.

Why Overwhelm?

So why are we overwhelmed? Here is a list of just a few of the things most coaches, whether marketing coaches or chiropractic coaches, tell us to implement.

Hold your breath, you'll be able to recognize some of this stuff...

New client welcome series, a welcome pack, social proof, indoctrination campaign, reminder texts, emails, phone calls, NFA procedure, dinner with the doc, orientation talks, screenings, screening scripts, screening teams, screening manuals, corporate talks, direct mail, postcards, Google reviews.

Pay-Per-Click, reports, Facebook talks advertising, Facebook views objectives, client appreciation events, referral campaigns, business cards, referral vouchers, email campaigns, reactivation campaigns.

CRM, front-desk software management, team meetings, front desk manuals, DC manuals, newspaper ads, editorials, guest writer, blogs, website, SEO, Twitter, Snapchat, Instagram, Facebook likes and check-ins.

Segmented campaigns, top three squeeze pages, videos, welcome pages, Yelp, workshops, events, surveys.

Maybe you'll feel a little overwhelmed already just reading that list. That's why we end up doing nothing.

For example, have you have ever been told that you should implement a marketing calendar in your business? I've been told that so many times.

But the calendars I've seen are very complex and if you tell me to try to implement all of the elements, it literally hurts my brain.

I have a full marketing team that cannot even come close to implementing it all. I find it very hard to believe that the people that suggest some of this stuff do it themselves or simply they are not running a practice anymore and have lost touch with reality.

Here's is an example of just the social media bloc of one calendar I recently saw:

- Facebook: 2-3 posts per day
- Twitter: 3 posts per day
- LinkedIn: 1 post per day
- YouTube: 1 post per week
- Google+: 2 posts per day
- Instagram: 1-2 posts per day
- Blog: 1 post per week

- Podcasting: 1 per week

- Pinterest: 1-2 posts per day

- Email: 1 per week

So, you're looking at anywhere from 10 to 15 social media posts a day. I ask you, what human being has ever done this type of thing consistently?

I promise that if you try implement EVERYTHING or every new marketing trend it will be very overwhelming... and end up implementing nothing...

Like I say, I've got a full team and there's really no way we can do this. What happens is we just end up being overwhelmed and opt out of doing anything at all.

I promise you that if you try to implement everything or every new marketing trend, it's going to be very overwhelming for you and then you're going to end up implementing nothing.

There's loads of stuff that I am going to talk about here, but I'll tell you that one of the keys to success for me is that I'm very good at focusing on three to six strategies that are my bankers. Do them well and do them consistently and the results will astound you.

I want to show you how to do that as well.

Why We Don't Do the Bankers

I truly believe that you will go through this book and there is going to be a couple of strategies you're going to learn that are going to absolutely change the game for you.

But there's also going to be a couple of strategies that you realize that you already knew, that you're just going to learn how to scale it or make it bigger. And that's where a lot of you will get your biggest breakthrough while reading this book.

The bankers I'm talking about are right under your nose. Many of them you've done but you stopped doing them because of a couple of things.

One of the reasons is that we often get bored. We just get bored of that one strategy. We don't know our numbers, so we don't actually know how good it is. And we end up looking for the next shiny object syndrome, like chatbots or the next awesome Facebook thing that comes out.

I've been there. It's like, "Wow, how cool is that? I can sit in my office and I can generate hundreds of leads without doing anything."

Often, it's just "one" strategy that will double your new clients... Often its right under your nose.

———

So, we get bored. We get shiny object syndrome, when we look at the next cool thing and we're ever hopeful that the next silver bullet is just around the corner.

We're going to cover a several strategies in this book, but I really want to stress this: Often it's just one strategy that will double your new clients.

I've seen it many times, there is often going to be just one that you rinse and repeat, or you literally scale up. It's often going to be one that's going to double your new clients.

Most of the time, it's right under your nose and I'm just going to help you with the nuances of that and you'll find this book is just a reminder.

You should be looking for the one thing in every chapter that you're really going to rinse, repeat and scale.

As we'll discuss, most people don't know how to scale an ad campaign because they don't know their numbers. They don't know whether it's working or not, and then they are not aware that they can actually spend more. So that's the first thing.

Ultimately, you'll be able to double, triple or quadruple your new clients with two or three strategies.

For this to work long-term, you're going to need multiple strategies.

———

The reason we learn more than one strategy is that the worst number in business... and you will quote me on this in the future, and this single thing will change your business in many respects... the worst number in business is ONE – one source of new clients, one client, one vendor.

The one thing might be a short-term win but to build a robust business, you need to function as if any one source could be taken away from you tomorrow.

And, trust me, any one of your sources of new clients can be taken away from you tomorrow and you still need to be in a position that enables you to grow.

That line right there has probably been the foundation for me setting up so many sources of new clients because one of the most lucrative sources of new clients could be taken away from me in a heartbeat.

When you try to feed the beast, especially having eight offices, it's a scary place, when you are heavily reliant on one major source of new patients. And I hated being in that position. So, I needed to become a master of creating multiple sources of new clients.

Avoiding Dead Time

In business, you cannot afford to have any what I call, "Dead time".

Dead time, refers to when you sit down to write that first marketing campaign or that first newspaper ad, and that first hour you are trying to put pen to paper and simply get going with not a clue how to start.

So, the biggest thing you'll get from this book is to decrease that start time or that dead time. I have throughout my career just bought that skill in many, many times.

Obviously, that's what you are doing here; one of the biggest things is you decrease overwhelm by reading this book. Because you'll be able to start the process so much quicker and that is really the key. The hardest thing is to start.

More than Marketing

Also, I'll just add one thing, whilst we're going to be focusing on marketing a lot in this book, the ultimate goal is for me to do everything in my power over the next seven chapters to help you with the following.

- Serve more people
- Make more money – it is a business after all
- Reproducible systems
- For some people, scaling up. For others, just one practice that's nice and big
- Multiple steams of new clients
- A better business with less stress and more time

So, as we go through this, I'm not only going to share the marketing strategies, I'll also share some key business, sales, team and life strategies.

Good News and Bad News

So, before we go on, there's good news and bad news. The good news is the stuff that I'm going to teach you works. I'm in the game. I know it works. We've still got lots to learn, trust me, but this stuff just works.

It's also simple. Anyone can do it.

But now the bad news. While it's simple, it's not easy.

There are no silver bullets. I've been looking desperately for almost ten years and it just doesn't exist.

I've paid marketing agencies… I once got a quote from a marketing agency for over $10,000 a month to marketing strategies for me. We settled on a three-month trial and I paid him $5,000 a month for three months. My marketing guy had just started and was 19 at the time. At one stage his results were so bad that I was convinced that with a little input from me, the 19 year old kid I had just hired would outperform any of there campaigns and that's exactly what happened. We literally outperformed them 50 to one and this guy is a really big name in the online marketing space.

While this is simple, it's not easy.
There are no silver bullets.

———————

So, there are no shortcuts. There is no agency that you can pay to save the day. Nobody knows your business and target market better than you and therefore you stand the best chance to make a success of creating a flood of new patients.

It's simple, but it's not easy and it's often a learning curve, especially with technology, but I will help you with that.

Sometimes you will have less time in the beginning while you are learning so that you can have more free time in the future.

Most importantly, it's definitely not always sexy. But my question to you is, are you OK with an unsexy business that serves more people, makes you more money and gives you more freedom?

Yes, you're going to have to implement some strategies and take action, but it works. And I'll teach you how to make it work for you. So, let's get started.

THE MARKETING FUNDAMENTALS

I find that a big mistake many people make in marketing is that they rush straight into specific marketing activity without understanding how it all fits together.

So, over the next couple of chapters, I'm going to go over some of the important fundamentals that can determine your success or otherwise in marketing. In this chapter, I'll cover:

- The true importance of marketing

- The mindset for marketing success

- Separating strategy from tactics

- Knowing the numbers

The True Importance of Marketing

I'll start by telling you about the first marketing conference I ever went to. I was about 25 and I flew all the way to the USA to listen to a guy I'll mention several times, because he's really been a big influence on me, and that's Dan Kennedy.

There were a thousand people in the room and he said, "Where are my chiropractors, dentists, doctors and physiotherapists?"

We put up our hands and he said, "I just want to tell you all that you are all the absolute worst to work with. Just nightmares."

And I was like, "Dude, I've just flown all the way from the UK to sit in this room. I've spent thousands of dollars doing this within my first year of practice. Are you serious?"

But what he was alluding to is that we struggle with the word "marketing," we struggle with the word "sales."

So, I really want you to understand that marketing is really just helping people find you and helping them come to a decision to use your service faster than they would normally left to their own devices.

Marketing is helping people "find" you and helping them come to a "decision" to use your service "faster" than they would normally.

That's all it is, just a process of helping people.

The first stage is helping prospects to become aware of you.

The next stage is helping them to make a decision to use your product faster than they would normally, by making a series of micro-commitments.

That's all marketing is. You just assume that they were all going to use your product or service anyway but left to their own devices it would take them, say 5 years to find you – or more likely they will find someone else first.

Ultimately, they are probably going to use someone to solve the problem they have. Your job is just to speed up the process between then fumbling around looking for someone and finding you.

This sentence I'm going to teach you now without a doubt changed my life. This is really the basis of this book and most of the things I do in life are already based on it.

Here it is: **"You will always influence or help more people by mastering the marketing and/or teaching of the thing as opposed to just the doing of the thing."**

I learned that from Dan Kennedy and the reason he said we're all a nightmare to work with is because as chiropractors we spend the majority of our time doing the thing, in this case adjusting and not spending enough time also working on becoming great marketers .

Of course, doing the thing i.e. adjusting is important, but you will always influence and help more people by mastering the marketing or the teaching of the thing as opposed to just the doing of the thing.

Now I don't really see a difference between marketing and teaching. As you know, the definition of doctor is teacher. So that's all I think I'm doing when I'm marketing.

Every success I've had is because I marketed hard enough and taught enough. At my practices, that's one of our slogans – we train our way to success.

So, training, teaching, marketing – they are really all the same.

Marketing Mindset

In order to succeed in marketing, we need to change our mindset and act differently.

In his fantastic book "Trust-Based Marketing," Dan Kennedy talks about some of the reasons why marketers fail, or businesses fail. This is a very, very important list.

Number one, unreasonable expectation regarding the necessary investment in customer acquisition.

The key word is <u>necessary</u> investment. How do you know how much you can invest?

We'll cover that in this book. If you walk away with just that one thing from this book, you'll have changed your business.

Next one on the list is inadequate preparation for sales appointments and presentations.

Are you winging it? How many times have you walked into a Report of Findings and you haven't looked at the new client notes, you're not familiar with what's going on. You haven't had enough time to prep those x rays.

Maybe you've had a challenging client just before you walked into a report of findings but you haven't taken the time to get into a new state to make sure you're ready for that client to serve them and be present with them.

Next is acting on assumptions. For example, if I ask my marketing team, "How did that campaign go?" they know the worst thing they can say to me is, "It was good."

Because "good" is not an answer. That's an assumption.

Why marketers fail
Dan Kennedy list...

- Unreasonable expectations regarding **necessary investment** in customer aquisition.
- **Inadequate preparation** for sales appointments and presentations i.e. winging it.
- **Acting on assumptions** rather than collecting verified factual information.
- Hastily creating advertising without research, tested and proven models, or copywriting skill **(developed or purchased)**.

So, acting on assumptions rather than connecting verified facts and information is a cause of failure.

Next problem is hastily creating advertising without research, tested and proven models or copywriting skills (developed or purchased).

I really want to stress that I have short-cut almost everything in this whole process of marketing because I bought in the knowledge wherever I could and it's certainly something that people don't do enough of.

These are clearly general points that apply to any business, so I created my own list of why chiropractors are struggling to market themselves.

Number one on my lists is overwhelm. I already spoke about that in depth, but it's a huge problem.

For example, looking at that marketing calendar I mentioned, and I know I'm harping on about this, I beat myself up for a while going, "Well, I'm pretty good at marketing, but I'm not doing half the stuff."

If I did that, then I am pretty sure you're doing it.

The next thing for me is practices don't understand what they can and need to spend to acquire a new patient. The key word is "can" not so much need. We've already talked about that and we'll go into more detail shortly.

Next is lack of consistency. I'm telling you, you're going to go through this book and there's one or two strategies where you're going to go, "I'm aware of that. I've done that. I did that pretty well. Why am I not doing it anymore?"

Why do practices struggle to market themselves... Ryan's list...

- **Overwhelmed**, don't know where to start!
- Don't understand what they **CAN** and **NEED** to spend to acquire new patients.
- Lack of **consistency**.
- **No measuring.**
- Not enough client aquisition **Channels.**
- Lacking adequate **retention** or **conversion.**
- Don't invest in **ongoing mentorship.**

It's one of those things, you got bored. But I'm telling you, if you're OK with having an unsexy business, then I'm the right person for you because I'm very good at being consistent.

The secret to success is just show up. I tell my clients all time, I'm not very good at much. I just out show-up, most people.

Next, most people don't measure what they do so they don't know what they're doing. We'll talk more about that shortly.

Next one is not enough client acquisition channels, which I'll help you with. You cannot have one. It's too stressful.

Lacking adequate retention or conversion. That's not really within the remit of this book but it's big. It costs 8 to 10 times more to get a new client as opposed to keep one or reactivate one.

Now here's the big one. People don't invest in ongoing mentorship. I truly believe this. There's some magic that happens just by you believing in yourself to invest in yourself.

At any one time, I'm part of three or four masterminds. People who do one-on-one work with me know it's pretty expensive. But I always feel very congruent when I tell someone how much I charge, because I know that I pay way more than that.

The single biggest challenge with working with chiropractors when it comes to marketing is the self-imposed fear from peer to peer judgments.

Honestly all human beings are simply poor performers left entirely to there own devices. I need the right people around me that will keep me accountable. As Tony Robbins very correctly says, "environment is always stronger than willpower".

The single biggest challenge with working with chiropractors when it comes to marketing that Dan Kennedy mentioned is the self-imposed fear from peer to peer judgments.

That's what he alluding to when he said we were terrible to work with because first, we don't like the words sales and marketing. But the other thing he said was, "You're so scared of what other people think of you, especially our fellow chiropractors."

We've all been there and I'm not immune to it either. I was sitting in a conference once and I heard this line and literally, every time I have any fear of implementation or doing something… and I do have fear often, I'm not immune to it… this single line always helps me just take action and do it.

If you want to be good at this thing called business and marketing, you have to understand this one thing. **The person that is prepared to look stupid in public more often than his competitors will win.**

I never forget hearing Richard Branson at an event once say, "If you're going to be in this thing called business or this marketing world, you have to be very OK with the fact that you're going to end up with a lot of egg on your face. And, the more egg on your face, probably the more successful you'll end up."

I'm not saying that you purposefully go out there to look stupid, but just keep in mind that one line because, I'm not going to lie, you're going to mess up. But if you've got the right attitude and you have the right support around you, you'll laugh about it.

It will always be bragging rights as to who messed up the most. "Oh, my word, what an idiot! I forgot to put the telephone number on 5,000 sheets that went out," but there's no other way to learn.

I promise you, that when your surrounded by the right people who are action takers and high achievers, it will be a competition of who messed up the most, a kind of bragging right. Within the right context, if you are messing up a lot, that means you're taking a lot of action, and probably that your on the right path.

Understanding the Difference Between Strategy v Tactics

Let's talk about strategies and tactics. Strategies will trump tactics every time, so most of what we will talk about here will be strategy not tactics.

A lot of stuff you're seeing in the market now is just a race to the bottom.

The implementation of strategy changes with the times a bit, but honestly, even at these massive conferences I attend with the best marketers on the planet, even when you meet with a few of the top marketers in private rooms, it is clear that a lot of stuff you're seeing in the market now is just a race to the bottom.

All this, "What bot can I implement, what new quick-win tactic can I do?" is just a race to the bottom because the old, time-tested strategies which we're going to cover will trump these quick-win tactics every time.

With that in mind, I can't begin this without teaching you this simple concept that was taught to me by Jay Abraham.

Anyone on my team will tell you that I regularly come back to this.

There are essentially only three ways to grow your business:

- Increase your number of new clients

- Increase the price

- Increase the number of transactions per customer
  (In chiropractic, we call this the PVA, the patient visit average)

We'll often come back to this in my business. We'll be stuck with how to break through a ceiling here in the business and I'll say, "Stop!" and put these three things on the board and ask, "What can we do?"

So, if you want 30 percent growth, all you basically need to so is increase your new patients by 10 percent, increase the price by 10 percent and you increased the number of transactions per customer (PVA) by 10 percent, you will actually increase your business by more than 30 percent.

We'll talk about strategies for these as we go through the book. But I want to start with a word about price.

I have started working with clients who are charging $100 for an adjustment and some who charge $50 and others who charge $30.

But it's also about habit and mindset.

When I'm coaching someone who's at $30 I say, "Just go to $40." If there action takers they go ahead and do it and they can't believe that it makes no difference to the amount of patients or visits they see weekly. Nobody leaves. It's all good. It's all our own fears around it that stop us from raising our prices.

So, here's a statistic that's going to put your mind at ease. If you raised your prices by 10 percent, and 20 percent of your patients decided to leave and never come back (never ever happened), you would still be on the same turnover or revenue as before the price rise.

When I tell people that statistic, it really puts their mind at ease and it helps people start to charge what they are worth or at least raise there prices by 10%.

Knowing the Numbers

One of the key fundamentals of marketing success is knowing the numbers in your business so that you can make the best decisions.

We'll look at several elements of that.

Measuring What Matters with Scorecards

This was a big game changer for us. It literally improved our business by 30 percent.

The single biggest failure I see in small to medium sized businesses is they don't measure what matters.

> ## ***Game changer alert***
>
> "What gets measured improves"
> The single biggest failure I see in businesses:
> Failing to know your numbers.
>
> Pearson's Law
> "That which is measured improves. That which is measured and **reported**, improves exponentially."

So, one thing that is important to understand is that what gets measured, improves.

But, here's the real game changer, Pearson's Law states that something which is measured improves, but that which is measured and reported on, improves exponentially.

The way we report what is measured is using scorecards.

I'm absolutely like a broken record with my team. If you want improvement, you'd better measure it and you'd better put it on a big whiteboard somewhere for everybody to see and make someone accountable for it.

Warren Buffett said, "If you can't read the scoreboard, you don't know the score and if you don't know the score, you can't tell if you're winning or losing."

Scorecards were made famous in business by Dan Sullivan of Strategic Coach. What Dan really helps people understand is really the five to 10 numbers you would need to see if you were stranded on a desert island somewhere and wanted to know the health of the business.

We've got many scorecards. It's key to have a measurement for each department – everyone has a number and there's one person responsible for making sure everybody gets their numbers.

Here are some of the things we measure on our scorecards, some you may not have thought of:

- Phone answer rate. You are throwing money away if the phone isn't answered. We've got a 95 percent answer rate goal and last week we were at 93 percent. I think it's massively important.

- Visits booked ahead of time. One of the biggest challenges is what they called the "stress of the sale". If you look at your diary and you've got a near capacity diary two weeks ahead you come from a different place in that you don't need to make that next sale. Necessity drives away opportunity.

- Average fee per visit. Some of you will be very, very surprised about how much did you actually make per visit? Even though your adjustment fee might be $50, $75, $100 with all the plans, what are you actually working at?

- Collections v Services: The difference between collections and services is taking into account plans that you sold and it's important to look at that. We set our targets on services but collections is important to know what money is coming into your business.

- Marketing Scorecard: We produce this every week covering number of leads, number of new clients, source of introduction. I need to know where they're coming from and then we go back and look at what is the most valuable source for us.

Scorecards can be spreadsheets, or they can be whiteboards on the wall. We have both for different purposes.

If you're feeling overwhelmed, I get you. Rome wasn't built in a day, but you need to be looking at this on a weekly basis.

If you just add your own scorecard from next week, you will change your business. I promise you.

Three Key Numbers

Many of the things we measure on our scorecards are important but, from a marketing perspective, there's really three numbers you need to know.

As I said earlier, if this is the only thing you walk away with from this entire book, you're going to understand some real sound marketing foundations.

First of all, you cannot market your business effectively if you do not know **Client Lifetime Value**.

> ## ***Game changer alert***
>
> **Key Marketing Stats**
> If you just know these three you will be
> in the top 2% in the profession
>
> • Your client lifetime Value (LV)
> • Cost per lead (CPL)
> • Cost per new client (CPC)

You need to be able to work out the lifetime value of a client that comes to you because it's a game changer for how you market your business, and in fact make just about any decision in your practice.

If you don't know this number, how can you ever tell how much you can "afford" to spend to acquire a new patient.

When you know your lifetime value, you may well realize you can spend way more, than your currently comfortable spending, to get a new patient.

The Easiest way to work out you approximate lifetime value of a patient, is to multiply you Patient Visit Average (PVA) by you average adjustment fee.

Let me go back one step. There is more than one way to approximate your PVA, the key is not to get too hung up on it but just to remain consistent with the way you finally settle on. The way we work out our PVA, is by calculating the total number of visits' in the diary (including New Patient Visits) over a 6 month period and dividing that by the total number of New Patients over the same time period. (Total visits / New Patients= PVA)

Once you have your PVA you simply multiply it by your average adjustment fee. Be wary to just use your pay per visit fee to do this if you have discounted care plans. The real average adjustment fee is usually lower than you may think when you take into account all discounts etc.

So for example if your PVA is 24 visits and your average adjustment fee across the board is $45 , then your Lifetime value would be $1080. (24x $45= $1080)

Next number is **Cost Per Lead.** Your cost per lead is what it costs you to move someone from just a person in the marketplace to a prospect. Strictly speaking, a "lead" is someone that has given us their contact details and/or you are in active "conversation" with that via various media.

So, how much does it cost you to get the contact details for each person?

That is quite different from the next number, which is even more important. This number is the **Cost Per New Client.**

Your cost per new client is what it actually costs you to get them into the clinic for an initial consultation or Day 1 assessment.

The difference between the two is that a "lead" is worked out by simply looking what it cost to get them to swap details vs Cost Per Client takes into account any additional expense it takes and/or any extra front end income that comes in from the lead going from "lead" to "New patient in clinic". For example it may cost $50 in advertising costs per potential client, to get that person to give us their details for a specific Facebook campaign (cost per lead). However that client may have opted in for a 50% offer that for example would require them to pay $50 dollars when they come into the clinic. Therefore on the front end it cost us zero to acquire that customer (cost per client). We will go into more detail in a moment.

From a marketing perspective, if you know those three, you're good.

ACTION STEP

Work out the Client Lifetime Value for a patient in your practice.

Why These Numbers Matter

Why it's important to know your numbers is because of this quote. This is the whole key to marketing: "The person that is willing and able to spend the most to acquire a new customer wins."

> ### ***Game changer alert***
>
> "The person that is **willing** and **ABLE** to spend the most to acquire a new customer, wins."

The key word is "able". That's why you need to know your numbers.

Without knowing lifetime value, you can never fully understand what you can afford to spend on marketing. This makes a marketing budget irrelevant.

Let's look at an example of why a marketing budget is irrelevant when you know the lifetime value of one of your clients.

- Let's say the lifetime value is $1,000.

- Can you afford to spend $100 to get a client with a lifetime value of $1,000. Of course you can.

- Can you afford to spend $200? Absolutely.

The reality is that 99 percent of chiropractors wouldn't dream of spending that much, but you can absolutely afford to do that.

Obviously you need to take into account operating cost etc. Also, bare in mind that, when you have associates, the margins are lower as you have to take into account associates' fees and again operating costs. In that case you usually can't "afford" to spend as much to get every new client.

Cost Per Lead v Cost Per New Client

Here is another example of the difference between the two. I've had some unbelievable campaigns on Facebook, where we've generated for example 80-150 leads.

Now to fully understand the difference between CPL and CPC just consider that some studies have shown that it can take 10-18 follow-up calls to get hold of them if ever at times, meaning that even though they have given you there details, they may never actually end up becoming a new patient. This is why robust follow up systems are important, and one of the first things we help my Inner circle members get implemented.

When I look at it, I might have got 80 opt-ins but I'm still in the process of getting them to come in. perhaps about 40 of them have actually come in for the appointment and in that case your going to have a substantially higher cost per client that cost per lead.

A lot of people show some very sexy stats on Facebook for example for cost per lead and record marketing campaigns.

I'm telling you now, without a follow-up system, especially with an answer rate of between 10 and 18 calls in some circumstances, a lead means nothing if you don't have some systems in place to follow up.

We'll talk more about that later.

Reducing Marketing Costs

When you are looking at your cost per new client, you have to consider the fact it's not just to get them into the examination.

Even in the first meeting, they may still be a prospect or a lead. They don't become clients until they pay.

Often the initial examination may be free (although its not necessary nor recommended), but all they have to do is pay for x-rays, if required, depending on how you practice.

But getting that payment for the x-ray really helps with marketing costs. That is what they call a self-liquidating offer.

You see this with offers online where once you've placed your order, you'll normally go to another page and they'll say, "Oh, by the way, I know you were interested in the 10 ways to look sexy and healthy. You might be interested in this $20 self-study book."

It's not a big offer. The only purpose of that offer is to decrease the marketing cost. So, they will drive you to another page where they get you to pay a small price for something.

At least 30 percent of people often do it. That's the way it works, and they really decrease their marketing costs.

You can think of it the same way when someone comes into your clinic, whatever your special was, whatever your cost per lead was, I want you to consider the fact that if you take any money from them at that initial examination … you can deduct that from the cost, and that's your actual cost per client.

Velocity of Return

Next number I want to talk about is one that nobody talks about in a business and it's going to kill your cash flow, and this is velocity of return.

This means if I spend $100 to get a client, how long does it take me to get that $100 back?

If you spend $100 and the client is paying $50 per adjustment, it's basically two or three adjustments and you've got all your money back and now you're in profit. That's a good thing.

But, especially if you spend more on marketing than most, the timing is important. Even though the lifetime value might be $1,000, if for example I have smaller margins, as is the case in an associate practice, from a cashflow perspective, its important to understand how long it may take to get that initial marketing investment back.

If for example you offer clients options to pay for a number of visits in advance, then your velocity of return will be very fast compared to someone who doesn't offer that option. There is no right or wrong but, its important to factor in when you are planning your marketing, in order to manage your cash flow responsibly.

That being said, we are very blessed in chiropractic, we have got a great profit margin, and in most cases, a great velocity of return. If you've got a high lifetime value, you can really dominate your market.

It's Not a Choice Between A or B

Now I just want to run through a scenario with you. Let's say you've got two sources of new clients and let's assume your lifetime value is $1,000

Let's assume one source of new clients has a cost per client of $25 and the other source of clients is $55. Which one are you going to do?

Many would say you're obviously going to do A instead of B.

But I want to be clear. It's not an "or" conversation, it's an "and" conversation.

You are going to do A and B. The fact that A is cheaper than B is irrelevant.

To this day, there are times I'll find myself at times going, "We're obviously going to do that one, right?" and then I just have to remind myself the fact that A is cheaper than B is irrelevant.

The correct question to ask is, "Do they both make sense when you look at lifetime value and cost per client?"

This is a little bit harder than you may think because I promise you, you're going to look at your cost per new client and you're going to think, "This one is so much cheaper, let's just do more of that."

I'm telling you right now. That will limit your scaling ability.

Successful people do not think "either/or," and I do not just mean this with marketing, this is also true in life. Successful people think both.

THE THREE KEYS OF MARKETING

There are three main elements you need to take into account in planning your marketing and we're going to look at each.

They are:

- **Market** – who is your customer?

- **Message** – what are you saying to them?

- **Media** – how do you reach them?

Let's look at each individually.

The Market

Most people approach their businesses as though they are desperate to get customers and they will be happy if anyone comes and gives them money.

Now I'm not saying you should turn people away potential customers. But I do say that your marketing will be easier and more effective if you know who you are going after.

So, my question to you is, who is your perfect customer? Who do you want to work with? Or, better yet, who do you already attract?

Now I'm going to be honest about this part. I struggled with it for years and I refused to do it.

Every coach I worked with made me do this. I hated it. I couldn't see the point of it.

I'd go from marketing consultant to marketing consultant and they all said to do this. I hated it until I "got it" and it was literally years I was fussing with this thing.

Every single consultant I spoke with said, "You've got to know your perfect client." At the time, it just didn't make any sense to me. But I can tell you, it is worth it.

It's going to help you:

- Plan your marketing activity more effectively

- Write better copy

- Attract the ideal people to your talks and events

I'm talking about clearly defining your ideal customer or creating what we call an "avatar". An avatar is simply a way of describing your ideal customer as if they were a specific person.

You've got two ways to work out what your avatar is:

- Demographic information

- Psychographic information

Demographic information is factual data such as where they live, their age, gender, education level, household income, marital status and occupation.

Psychographic information is more about how they think and behave. It is their opinions, values, personality type or their lifestyle choices. It can also be their hobbies, the magazines they read, what shops they hang out in, what brands they wear or their religious beliefs.

There's a famous story about a business owner who completely transformed his marketing based on this. He sent out a questionnaire to his clients and asked them various questions, including what magazines they read.

Lo and behold, he discovered that 70 percent of his clients read the same specific magazine.

So where do you think he advertised? In that magazine, of course. It changed his business. So, this is important stuff to know.

In my business, we actually have three avatars. We have more than 30 chiropractors and cover a range of markets and areas. So, for us, three avatars is a necessary evil.

For most practitioners, I'd say one is enough at least until you get started and you can add others later.

By sharing the three with you, I hope it helps by giving you a broad range of examples rather than scaring you by making it look too complicated.

All of the avatars have a name to make it as real as possible. You might even find it helpful to use a picture, whether a model or a real person.

Halsa Avatars – Fiona

- 35 – 65, female
- Middle class
- With pain or with family members in pain
- Wants convenience – we're the last resort, just wants to be helped
- Previous treatment failed, will do whatever it takes
- Little stress
- Wants credibility and social proof
- Family friendly
- Located – Thames Valley: 3–4 miles, London: 1–2 miles

Our first avatar is Fiona, 35 to 65-year-old female, middle class with pain or with family members in pain.

She wants convenience. Often, we're the last resort, but she just wants to be helped. Previous treatments failed so she will do whatever it takes.

She wants little stress. She wants credibility and social proof.

She wants to go to the best and a family-friendly place. I personally love dealing with these clients.

Next is Bob, a 25 to 55-year-old male, physical worker – a labourer, a tradesman.

Halsa Avatars – Bob

- 25 – 55, male
- Physical worker/labourer/tradesmen
- Cash-in-pocket
- Health is their pay-cheque – want to get sorted to get back to work
- Lost income due to pain
- Plays sports at weekend

Many of us have had these amazing clients like a window cleaner or a bricklayer or a roofer.

They get cash in hand, they're self-employed and if they don't work, they don't earn.

Their health is their paycheck so they need to get back to work.

Clients like these are really good for retention because they might lose income due to pain. They generally play sports at the weekends.

Halsa Avatars – Harvey

- 35+
- Desk-bound
- Corporate environment
- Office workers
- Educated in health
- Proactive about their health
- Stressed

The last one is Harvey, your corporate person, aged 35+, desk-bound, corporate office environment. Educated about their health, proactive about their health and stressed.

Those are our three avatars. Best way to start this is by describing someone you currently see or a specific demographic you currently see a lot in the practice or just like seeing.

Who do you love to see? It's just a dream to work with them. You don't lose any energy when you're with him or her. That's the way you want to be looking at this.

ACTION STEP

Create an avatar for your ideal client

For me personally, it was like your slightly older lady, 50+ who lived in the area, disposable income, really sweet and you'd always have a laugh and a joke with them. That was my perfect client. So, choose one.

The Message

The next key element is the message. We'll be talking about the messaging more specifically in later chapters but, at this stage, I want to address one specific white elephant in the room, and that is "pain". People often get this upside down and think that because for example they are a "vitalistic" chiropractor, they should in no way mention "pain" in their marketing.

All I can say… and this was taught to me very early in my career… **"pain is the doorway to wellness"**. If there was no pain, chiropractic would have a very tough time being where it is now.

> ## Pain is the doorway to wellness care…
>
> Give them what they want so that you can educate them as to what they can have over time…
> The miracle of chiropractic
>
> BJ Palmer himself said, SYMPTOMS SELL

I'm on board with the importance of wellness but you have to understand you need to, "give them what they want, so that you can educate them as to what they can have over time"… and that is the miracle of chiropractic.

I have been through this emotional battle in my head many times, but this really changed things for me. B J Palmer himself said, "Symptoms sell."

You've got to be okay with that so that you can meet them where they're at, so you can take them to where they can be. I promise you it'll change your business.

The key to this whole thing is the customer is the hero. We are just the guide.

If they want to know more about their back pain, you give them that. If they want to know more information about their sciatica, give them more information about their sciatica. We are not trying to fit them in our box. The customer is the hero, we are just the guide.

However, it's also important to understand is that people do not come to see you because of pain. You may think they come to see you because the pain. They do not.

They come to see because the pain has affected their life at that point in time and stopped them from doing something. That is it.

Your job in the initial consultation and Report of Findings is to find out what that is. What is the real reason?

There are a few formulas for marketing, especially copywriting. One of them is – Problem, Agitate, Solve.

That means you find the pain and then you agitate or illicit it and then offer a solution. Let me give you an example. If someone says, "I can't get out of bed in the morning." An example of "agitate" is simply what most of us would regard a "caring" or "empathy by asking, "Oh wow, that must be really frustration, How does it affect your life?". They may respond with, "I'm really worried that it's going to get worse …" etc., etc.

A great phrase to repeat is, "Tell me more".

Here's the thing, you remember the cliché that the definition of "doctor" is "teacher." The word education comes from a Latin word to educe, meaning that you're not shoving information down anyone's throat. Educe means to draw out. That is your job. This is something we cover in depth with my inner circle clients at their live meeting (3 per year).

So, when you are thinking of your avatar, I really want you to think about what's their pain? What's the phrase they say when they go, "I just had to do something about this? For example, "I knew it was bad but when I couldn't pick up my daughter, I just knew I needed to do something.

Without that, it's very, very difficult to move someone along the buying process. Because the sales process is about them subconsciously justifying it to themselves.

Human nature is that we will do way more to avoid pain than to go towards pleasure.

Just think about the times you have maybe under played the severity of a certain problem a patient is suffering from and in doing so they may say something like "Oh wow, so I'm actually really good." In a Report of Findings. Its normally very difficult to get any compliance in patient care after that.

The reason for that is that people will make decisions based on two things – towards pleasure or away from pain. Towards pleasure is very difficult to "sell" or said differently it hasn't been done all that successfully in any market place, neither has "prevention".

Human nature will simply do way more to avoid pain, than to go towards pleasure. So, in your consultation and Report of Findings, you need to consider this.

Even in "How to Win Friends and Influence People," it says, "To be interesting, be interested." That's all you're doing is being interested. I want to be clear here, if you truly want to help people, by getting them enrolled in what I truly believe is the best health care product on the market, your job is simply to make every effort you can to find out the "pain" that is there and already exists. You are not creating pain, simply shining a light on the pain, fears and concerns that already exist. In essence you're a "truth finder".

Media

Let's now move on to the third key element, which is media.

As we get into the later chapters, where I teach you the New Patient Avalanche Blueprint, we'll be talking about specific media in more detail, including how to use them. So, for now, I just want to paint a big picture of the different options.

These days, there are so many things that you could be doing in your marketing. If there was ever an industry where we are susceptible to "shiny objects syndrome," it's marketing.

In our marketing room, we have to rein ourselves in big time – this new bot and this sexy thing here and there's lots of different media out there. So, I'm going to run through the big picture now, and then I'm going to break down, what I believe has been a winning formula for us.

Media can be split into three main categories – online, offline and live. All are important and we'll be going through how to make use of each but let's start with an overview.

Facebook

First in the online category is Facebook. We'll go into great detail on how I suggest you use Facebook later but there are many different ways you can use it.

Different options for using Facebook include, Facebook Messenger, lead generation, one-touch, two-touch, retargeting and custom audiences amongst many more.

One of the lead generation options is doing a Facebook ad and driving people to your blog. Now on the blog, you have something called the Facebook pixel so that you can "retarget" them. That means that if someone lands on that blog, you can retarget them with a different message on Facebook that only those people see within their news feeds.

You've probably seen it where you look at a website and all of a sudden you see their stuff in your Facebook feed. They do that with the Facebook pixel.

Other options on Facebook are that you can drive them to download a report or to interact in a quiz.

You can also have one-touch campaigns, where you're driving people to an initial consultation. However, I don't care how many people will tell you they can get 15 million leads with one-touch campaigns. You cannot rely on them only, because you will suffer from ad fatigue.

One of the most challenging things about our industry is that we've got tiny audience sizes. The experts on Facebook now are teaching that you need at least a million people in your audience to do it very successfully.

We've got, if we're lucky, 10,000-50,000 people in our audience sometimes, so you cannot be hitting that relatively small audience with a "Come for a special appointment" message over and over and over.

It may work once, but then you will reach ad fatigue and that's why you've got to have your two-touch campaigns.

That's where you're driving people to Facebook and they view a video, "10 Things You Can Do in San Diego Without Back Pain." Then you're going to re-target people who watched a certain amount of that video.

Then you've got retargeting and custom audiences. For example, if you have a list of people that haven't been in to see you for three months, what we do is we'll put them through a reactivation campaign. What we do is take the list… people over 18, had at least one adjustment, hadn't seen you, let's say for three months… and then you go back one year and two years and build the list.

Now you export that list and you put that into Facebook. Those people see a specific message. Let's say it's your Easter reactivation campaign. You can literally go, "Hey, have you got my email" on Facebook?

This is really cool and you don't have to pay that much because it's such a small audience. You can reach just the people that you want. You can do a custom audience just for your database so only they see it.

You could quite literally wave your newsletter and go, "Hey, make sure you check your emails. There's a newsletter, in your inbox."

So that's custom audience. Remember a key part of this whole book is just making you aware. It's like when you're thinking about buying a car and you really like one and then all of a sudden you see that car everywhere.

Now that I've said the word pixel, now that I've said the word custom audience, you are going to see those words everywhere.

Because of that, you're going to go from unconscious incompetence, to conscious competence. That's the point of this book. You've just gone from unconscious incompetence which is state of "not knowing what you don't know", to conscious incompetence. This is essentially an awareness that there is something to learn or as some would say "knowing what you don't know" and that is a learning opportunity.

For example, "Crap, I don't know anything about pixels and I don't know anything about custom audience."

Now, you're going to see it everywhere and you're going to watch a two-minute video or you're going to go to YouTube and you're going to click on "What is a pixel?" and you can have pixels going straight away. My Diamond member inner circle client for example get a full library of all the "how to's", but first they need to "know what they don't know".

Websites

Let's talk about websites. The only real purpose for your website is lead generation. Remember there is only a limited amount of things that you can focus on, specifically if you are practicing full time.

So, for me, I pay someone to do my website. I pay them a monthly fee. It really isn't that much, and I just get it out in my mind.

The only real purpose for your website is lead generation.

However, I can tell you, one year, we easily spent $50,000 on a website and it was the biggest waste of money ever.

All I really want to do is get my page to number one or number two in the search rankings. That's really all you need. There's so much to focus on that, for me, if I'm number one on organic search, I'm happy.

I'm not a guru with websites but I do think one thing you need to know is that your webmaster or whoever designs your website will not understand the concept of lead generation, which we will discuss shortly.

They'll think you're crazy, "Why do you want all these things?" Just tell them to shut up and say, "Look, I want lots of options for lead generation. I want 'click here for free consultation.' I want five reports. I want lots of options for lead generation."

They will argue with you, just tell them to trust you. They'll need your guidance.

Live Chat

Another thing is that live chat has been a big one for us. It's really cool. That's the way the world's working now. We book lots of people via some form of live chat, including Facebook live chat, which is huge at the moment, and I will teach you a little bit more about that.

You could turn it on during work hours, turn it off during non-work hours or you just have a basic bot on there that makes it look as if you've got a person at the live chat, but when it says, "How can I help you?" it replies, "I'm sorry, there's no one here right now. Please leave your email address and I'll get back to you." Again, that's just lead generation.

In my opinion, that's all a website is there for. You'll get very different views on this. But there is only a limited amount of things you can focus on. So, I just pay someone to do this for me and it's not a lot of money.

Pay per Click

Nobody can debate that ppc and google are powerful arsenals to be working for you and your marketing efforts. However that being said, you should know the following facts. Statistically, google spend more money "offline" than "online"

The online giants still take the time to send you a letter and phone you.

Google sell pay-per-click and they are an online business yet almost every business owner I know can attest to the fact that they have, at some point in their business careers, received a sales/promotional letter from Google selling pay per click or a phone call?

Just take a second to understand the above fact. The online giant, google, still take the time to send you a letter and phone you. They're selling you the once thought, "holy grail" of marketing, but they're not using their own pay per click to sell it to you. Anybody else see the irony in that?

Video

Now, let's look at video – Facebook Live, video in email, and Facebook Views Objective.

Video is a very important part to your marketing story. Its been said, that if you are not doing video on facebook, you don't exist

An interesting side note is that, at the time of writing this book, Green screen videos are being significantly out performed by "selfie" style videos. The selfie video is getting as much as seven to ten times more views than a "professional" green-screen video.

You can also easily put a custom video in email and GIFs are a big thing in emails at the moment to get open rates up.

The above information is not necessarily "news" to most reading this book but in my experience actually doing the videos is a "fear" for a lot of docs. This is good news for you, because by doing anything (no matter how bad" , you will set yourself apart from the "crowd".

Email

Let's talk about email. First of all, is email dead? I can absolutely tell you that email is not dead.

The big benefit of email is that it's one of the only media that you own.

Essentially the concept of the lead has changed. You can develop what they call a vertical on Facebook which is essentially, all those people that view your videos, you actually don't need their details anymore for them to be in your audience, because the power of Facebook is that you can easily retarget people that watch things or click on things.

The online giants still take the time to send you a letter and phone you.

But you can lose your Facebook account at any time. Facebook can kick you off. I've seen it happen many times to people and you lose all that hard work. Email is still probably the only media you own. You own that email list.

I promise you, we just don't send enough emails. It's as simple as that.

Every single time you send an email, you get clients, even if it's just planting a seed. If you have a call to action, every single time you send an email you make "money".

How much is too much? People are desensitized to emails these days because people opt in to so many things and people are sick and tired of so many things landing in their inbox.

Open rates have gone down. But when a top online marketer I follow was asked about this, he simply said, "I just send more. If it goes down further, I just send double".

I know you're freaking out right now. But I promise you, none of us, me included, are sending enough emails.

The key though is empathy and value in those emails. Most of the time, they don't even open them, so I don't know why we're freaking out about it.

I'll give you a formula for that later and I'll give you the easiest way that really helped me with my copywriting for an email that I sent that got 30 new clients in one email. It took me five minutes to write. You're going to love this when I teach it to you.

I'm going to teach you something called the "weekly nothing" email. That's the email that I sent that got 30 new clients, from one email.

The more you talk to your list, the more you can talk to your list. If you've never sent your list an email in 10 years and all of a sudden you start sending 30 emails a week, that's the shock to their system and maybe then you will have people opting out and complaining but for the most part, buy not sending regular communication via email is a big mistake I see all too often.

Print

One of the things I get asked a lot is, "Print advertising, newspapers, do they still work?" Absolutely. They still work.

However, don't personally do that much newspaper advertising. That is not to say that its not a very viable media for you but you will need to watch your velocity of return with this media as the cost per lead tends to be higher. Of course if your comfortable that your velocity of return is fast then this may be a real winner for you because often the quality of the lead can be higher.

I'm not going to go into this in detail because I don't do much of it anymore. I can get more leverage in other ways.

I am not a fan of magazines. However, I will tell you that there is one little niche that is just the most fantastic thing you can ever do.

We've done so well from this one little niche and it's your local publications, your Church magazine, those "Round and About" local community publication. The more amateur looking the better.

Some can be as little as $25 a month to advertise in. It's unbelievable. I still look at the stats to this day and cant believe how well they can work".

Because what happens with those local church/local-type publications is there is a huge amount of trust with that.

The fancy laminated magazine that all the reps are chasing you guys for, I've had very little traction with those.

Newsletters… have you ever tried a print newsletter before? Did you get frustrated with it? I know I have.

But, I'm going to tell you now, that they are an absolute hidden diamond. Yes, it takes some effort to put it together. But, in today's society, somebody goes home with a newsletter, it lies on their kitchen table, it goes on the fridge.

It has got one of the highest readerships and the longest time value, meaning it stays around in someone's house longer than any other media.

Newsletters are an absolute hidden diamond.

A letter, they read, and they chuck away; a newsletter normally lies around the house for days or weeks. I've got newsletters lying everywhere in my house.

For a newsletter, there's two options. You can hand them out to save costs, but it's really the people that aren't seeing you that need the newsletter.

Direct mail, you can massively bump response rates. They are normally secondary to an email or Facebook campaign.

If you can send them print media at some point in the campaign, it massively increases your response rates.

Postcards are still powerful, same as direct mail, posters and flyers.

Now let me say this, you can quote me on this. This is a Ryan-ism, nothing has ever been solved by a flyer in the history of mankind. No poster has ever saved a business. No flyer has ever saved a business.

The only reason anyone hands out flyers at a screening, is because they don't know what else to do.

Rather capture leads, capture leads, capture leads. Stop handing out flyers. They suck.

Get rid of all the flyers at your front desk basically. When somebody comes in, have an awesome looking picture of an amazing e-book and say, "Let me send you this."

That is probably the first place that people get traction when they start coaching with me is that concept.

When the person comes in and wants to know more, say, "Awesome, give me your email address and I'll send you everything you need to know."

That's what you do. You do not give them a flyer with prices in it.

Live Events

Live events, we've got screenings, talks in-house, talks in the community, talks in companies.

I want to just say the big thing with live events that nobody factors in is sometimes your return on investment can't be measured. Because what most people don't factor in is what it does to a community.

There is no substitute for changing the selling environment. There's no substitute for meeting live.

Just think of this. The concept that 5,000 online marketers fly all the way to San Diego to one of the biggest online marketing events in the world every February to meet in person is ridiculous if you think about how all those people do everything online.

There's no substitute for meeting live.

But there is no substitute for meeting in person, there's no substitute to getting people in a room and that is actually more of a retention strategy than anything.

I just want to state that the effect of live events, the effect of changing that environment is so important to the whole journey.

The traction that you'll get from your appreciation events, etc, is very important. A lot of the docs that I've coached, just that alone has increased their PVA.

The Growing Importance of the Conversation

Those are basically the media that we're going to run through but first I want to take a look at where marketing is going. This is a view of how things will develop.

The conversation is the new "lead". Everything we're doing in our marketing department is about how do we stimulate conversation? We're just about to do this, we're going to send an email and give them four options to respond to us.

The conversation is the new lead.

This goes straight to a Facebook messenger chat, Live Chat, bots, all those things, but it still just starts a conversation. The conversation is the new lead.

We often have great examples of this that proves this point beautifully below. Great ad on Facebook and someone just asks a question in the comments, and we replied, "Thanks for connecting. Here's a report that might answer your question."

She downloaded the report, but she did not email us back nor did she even look at the report but she continued that chat on Facebook messenger and there was a whole conversation. Towards the end, she just said, "How much will this cost?" and, when told the price, she said, "Awesome. Can I please book?"

So, the conversation is the new lead and it's really using automation and certain ways to get that into a one on one conversation.

We are moving more towards specific journey attention. I teach event-based marketing. We are even transitioning a little bit more to, as opposed to doing your Easter campaigns and Christmas campaigns, though we still do that, it's more based on going, "Hey Mary, I noticed you haven't been in in 30 days, just wanted to touch base and see how you doing?" . Continually stimulating conversation.

BUILDING A SYSTEM TO TURN LEADS INTO PATIENTS

Studies have shown that most people are just not ready to buy from you when you first interact with them, and this brings me to what we like to do, which is called Lead Generation Marketing.

According to Wikipedia, lead generation is: *"The initiation of consumer interest or enquiry into products or services of a business."*

A lead is usually allotted to an individual to follow up on. Once the individual (e.g. salesperson) reviews and qualifies it to have potential business, the lead gets converted to an opportunity for a business. The opportunity then has to undergo multiple sales stages before the deal is won."

These stages can be viewed as follows:

- Creating Funnels

- Building Bridges

- Following up

Creating Funnels

One definition of marketing is "progressively moving towards doing business with you by a series of *micro-commitments*."

It may start with someone seeing your marketing and going, "I'm really interested in that. I would like more information."

By asking for more information, they are making their first micro-commitment and they then become a lead.

The lead then becomes a prospect when they come into your office or they book an appointment.

The prospect becomes a client once they start care with you.

In marketing, this process is often described as a "funnel" and is illustrated on the chart on the right.

It's important to understand this process:

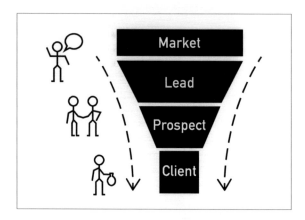

■ Your message goes out to the whole **market or a selected market**.

■ Someone shows interest in what you offer and they become a **lead when they share their contact information with you.**

■ They take that interest on further and become a **prospect when they decide to come into the practice for an initial appointment.**

■ The prospect comes into your business and goes through a sales process (Initial consult and report of findings) and then you have a **client/patient**.

To start this process off, you need to create a low risk way for potential customers to interact with you and you must make it easy for them to take a series of micro commitments towards your product or service.

When you look at the diagram, the market end is where it the interaction someone has with you needs to be low-risk.

We often underplay what a big financial and time commitment it is for someone to come into your office for your initial examination when essentially they don't know you from Adam.

What's the most precious commodity on the planet? It's time. Forget about the money. They probably spend about two hours in total between the journey their and the exam and in most cases they have never met you before. This cant be helped all the time but the point is to try be, omnipresent as Jay Abraham puts it. Meaning that by the time they walk into the office they have seen your face in multiple places (Facebook, newpaper , direct mail etc etc).

This Is why I am a big advocate not adjusting on the first visit. It allows you slow down the buying process and create a situation where you are positioned as the person that is giving the "solution". There are many sales and marketing books that speak about the first interaction being a 2 step process. That is essentially our Day one and Day two.

So based on that I would recommend not adjusting on the first visit. I know that's a big challenge for some of you, if you are doing it and you've heard it a million times.

After 10 years of working with docs and associates, I can tell you, simpy by looking at a few statistics who is adjusting on the first visit. The number one thing I find is that their PVA (patient visit average) will almost always be lower. You don't have to tell me their name, just from the statistics I can tell you who's adjusting on the first visit just because of the statistical effect.

We need to be thinking more "coffee on the first date" and not you know what.

You've got to have this process that's a series of micro-commitments that you're taking people through. Often people are just not ready to buy from you when you want them to. It has to be series of micro-commitments.

There is a time and place to go for the "sale". But I truly believe that we are way too "all or nothing" in chiropractic. We need to be thinking more "coffee on the first date" and not you know what.

In order to do this, you need to have adequate ways to follow up via a Customer Relationship Management system (CRM) or email system or at least manual call logs.

If you don't have a CRM or email system like Aweber, Infusionsoft or MailChimp, you need to get that sorted soon.

My CRM has made me hundreds of thousands of dollars just by sending the right messages at the right time.

A robust CRM can send texts, emails and mail and it even helps us with our Facebook campaigns and lead generation from a lead page and even systems such as Eventbrite sync with it.

Building Bridges

One of the easiest ways to start a relationship with a potential client is offer them "Information" in exchange for them giving you their contact details so that you can send it to them. This is called education-based marketing.

This is very key. Information is the bridge that helps people make decisions.

Now, I don't mean when they walk in, giving them a pamphlet at the front desk. That does not count because you don't have their contact details.

One of the quickest ways to get traction is when someone comes in and makes an enquiry, instead of giving them a pamphlet, get their email address and say, "I'm going to send you an information pack on everything that you need to know."

You can even have it laminated at the front desk and you can say, "I'm going to send you the 17 things you need to know before you choose a chiropractor."

> ## Information is the BRIDGE that helps people make a decision
>
> Your job is to create more bridges.

That's completely reasonable and you can email it to them right now. Now that person become a "lead". When you passively give them a pamphlet, and let them leave, you have completely lost control over having any effect on the outcome. Remember that marketing is simply the process of helping someone use your service faster that they would have, left to their own devices.

Information is the bridge that helps people make decisions. Your job is to create more bridges.

Studies show that if you don't offer information, people will want it before they are happy to use your product or service.

However, if you offer "information" , the prospect will often skip the information altogether and go directly to purchasing the product or service. So its not so much about how "good" the information is, it seems that research would suggest having "any" information is important.

Human beings are really bad at making decisions, so our default is to look for excuses as to why we can't make a decision.

Your job is to is to create a very low risk environment.

It should be no problem, "I'll give you my email address."

I know some people are hesitant to even give you their contact details, but it's still low risk as opposed to coming in and paying say $100 for an appointment.

Your job is to think "dating" as opposed to "I want to close the deal right now."

You're going to swap contact details for valuable information, and then you have a CRM built in to have a series of follow ups. It's a series of pre-identified ways to get people in and take them through the process.

If you're doing at least that, it's going to double your conversations. You've always got to have mixed media to get the best results, so don't just email them… send them a text, phone them and send them a piece of mail in the post, where possible.

Forms of Bridge

As I said, your job is to create lots of bridges. So, let's get into what a bridge is.

A bridge is a free report, like, "Seven Ways to Decrease Headaches Without Drugs or Surgery in Record Time."

There is no better bridge than a book. There's no better form of information and it's the best business card on the planet. We should all have a book at the front desk. But that takes some work so it's usually not the best place to start.

Coming to a health talk is also a bridge. It's a low risk environment. They come to a health talk, get to know you a little better and then there's an offer and we take them through a series of processes.

Coming to a Report of Findings as a guest is also a bridge. I'm actually not a huge fan of that but it is a form of low-hanging fruit where someone brings a family member. It's none threatening.

Forms of Bridges

- Free report
- Book
- Health talk
- Come to a RoF as guest
- Free offer
- Free telephone consultation
- Cost enquiry
- Free dowload
- Online Quiz

A free offer is a bridge, "Come in for a discovery session, a taster session and we'll tell you what's going on." There's no price, no fee and no obligation. We just tell you what's going on.

Free telephone consultations can be a great bridge. We have this on our website and it almost never ends up in a "free telephone consultation. Let me be clear, I, just like you, don't want to do free telephone consultations but when somebody fills this out they are clearly looking for some help. We get the front desk to call them and they almost always end up booking directly into a consultation before ever doing a "telephone consult". You see that's the point. At the time, for that individual it just seemed too much of a leap to pay for an examination but after hearing a friendly voice on the other side of the phone that cared, they felt just that bit easier about taking a "risk" to book an appointment.

Cost enquiry is the next one. Your website should never show your fees. Your job is not to answer all their questions, your job is to create questions. So, if you've given all your fees on the website, they don't have any need to phone you or enquire or email.

Other bridges are free downloads and online quizzes. People love quizzes. We do quizzes on Facebook all the time and the results are amazing. Once someone fills out a quiz on say "sciatica severity survey", they will be asked for there email address to send them the results. The stats are quite staggering. They show that if someone fills out the questionnaire and leaves there contact details, 80% and over will end up in an initial exam if our follow up phone call etc happens timeously.

This is a form of a bridge that we use regularly. It's an invite on Facebook to "Attend a FREE workshop, with limited availability, to help you safely and effectively manage headaches and migraines. Quickly book yourself in, and tag someone who needs this."

So that's a form of a bridge. It's free. We can have between 10 and 70 people register with an 80% show up rate if you know what your doing. Once in your office, if the correct processes are followed you can easily convert 80% of the attendees into a initial consultation.

If you looked at my website, you'd notice how many opportunities someone has to interact with me – they can click on "50% off," there's a web form, the free consultation, a phone consultation etc etc etc.

One of the easiest ways to create a "bridge" is to offer the option to download a free report on topics such as headaches and migraines, quick and easy ways to end back pain and stiffness, pregnancy related back pain and pelvic pain etc etc.

These are all free reports that we offer on our website and sometimes on facebook and we get hundreds of people downloading them every month. Every single day we get opt-ins. Think about it. People land on most websites and they just leave.

We often get over 40-60 people download our reports every week. Not bad for doing nothing extra. But now I've got the information, so now I can do something about it. FOLLOW UP and if need be offer another "bridge" if someone not ready to book an appointment. It's very powerful.

One of our free reports is "A Natural Way to Stop Annoying, Daily, Debilitating Headaches and Migraines from Disturbing Your Sleep, Mood and Daily Activities."

This is the page where we promote it.

A lot of people get freaked out by, "Oh, how do I make it look good?" Just go to www. fiverr.com and you can get someone on there to do that for you, no problem. You give

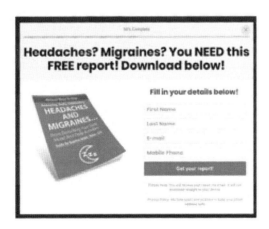

them the headline and they'll do that. We also cover this in depth in our New patient Avalanche course.

When they click to download the report, they go to an opt-in page.

To do this, you can get this built out by your website guy or use software like Lead Pages or Click Funnels, which will both get the job done.

So once they have clicked on the page, they will be given an option to fill in their name, last name, email and mobile number. And then we send them the report.

Then they get an automated email with the download saying, "Thank you very much for downloading our free report." There's no mention of a sale. It just has the valuable information.

Creating a Report

What goes in a report?
What would you tell your Aunty on the phone

Rules
Must take no longer than 30 min to write
Must take no longer than 10 min to read

Then we call them and simply say that this is a courtesy call to see if they received the information they requested ok. Then a well trained assistant will simply continue to ask questions and really show that they care by asking questions about what it was that was bothering them to download the information. This opens up dialog and often ends up in the person booking an initial consultation or another bridge such an a free informational talk.

I want to say one thing about creating the reports. What goes into them is exactly what you would tell your aunty on the phone. Really that simple.

You've all had this conversation before. Your grandmother phones you or your aunty phones you and says, "Oh, my word, my back's really sore what must I do?"

What are you going to say on the phone? That is exactly what you put in the report. The rules for this are it must take no longer than 30 minutes to write and it must take your clients no longer than 10 minutes to read.

If it takes you any longer than 30 minutes to write, you're not getting the point of this. Here's the thing… I promise you, they're probably not going to read it.

You might be thinking, "Why do I need to write it if they're not going to read it?" Ninety percent of them won't read it. But remember, if you don't offer information, they want it. If you do offer information, they often go straight to your offer.

The Fortune is in the Follow Up

One of the keys to the new patient avalanche is remembering that the fortune is in the follow up. I told you that this system works, but it takes work, and the fortune is in the follow up. I literally lost at least $350,000 on one marketing source by having poor follow up systems.

There was one source of new clients we were doing really well from. They actually had already paid for an appointment and I just assumed because they had paid for appointments that they were definitely going to come in, so maybe I didn't have to measure them so much. But you know what they say when you assume things – it makes an 'ass' out of 'u' and 'me'!

There were 1,500 new patients that I wasn't measuring. I measured getting them as clients, but I never measured whether they actually came in because they all paid up front for the appointment and therefore I slacked on my follow up and boy did I pay for it. So, over a couple years, there were 1,500 new clients who paid for appointments who didn't come in because my follow-up wasn't right.

It's at least $350,000 by the way, because let's say only 50 percent of them would have converted at just 12 adjustments, let's say at $50 each. That mistake cost me more than $350,000.

Now, the reason I bring that up is because remember, I'm in the business of making as many mistakes as quickly as possible.

And, I will tell you, if it's happening in my business, it's happening in your business, without a doubt.

As a ratio, it's exactly the same in your business. You're missing out on thousands of dollars because of the lack of follow-up in some way, shape, or form.

So here are the keys to doing this campaign successfully.

You've got to be tenacious. The answer rate on the phone can be as low as 1 in every 10 to 18 calls before they answer.

Now, the reason I lost $350,000 was because my procedure at the time stopped calling them after three tries which was way too early, hence we never got them booked in.

I recently saw a report by HubSpot this week saying that the normal average number of times you have to call someone before they answer is 18.

I personally know that I don't answer the phone when I don't know the number, and you probably don't either, so you've got to be more tenacious. That means they go on a spreadsheet or CRM and they stay on there until you get a hold of them.

The Fortune is in the FOLLOW UP...

Our call mistake that cost us 250k
Key points to do this successfully

- Be tenacious (Answer rate on phone is 10-18 times before they answer)
- Need a Script
- Track stats and call history
- When using Mobile to call - don't leave a message
- When using Landline to call - can leave a message
- Mix it up, Mobile and Landline
- Offer another BRIDGE
- Be prepared to "date" (CRM)

It doesn't matter if they say no, but they stay there until you get hold of them. That mistake cost me over $350,000.

Next you need a script that someone works through. All you're doing is phoning to see if they got the report safely.

By the way, there are other leads where people have opted in for an appointment and then it's the easiest call ever. This is a bit different. This is, "Hey, I'm just making sure you got the report. Oh, you asked for the back-pain report, Shane, what's going on?"

Then you just let them talk. Now, whoever is doing the calls has got to have empathy and they're going to feel that.

So, if you're good at this, you'll get an 80 percent conversion. If you're not so good at this, you get a 30 percent conversion which can make all the difference in your business.

So, it's simply a call and you've got to be OK with wherever they are. It's simply a call to find out what's going on. They will often talk the hind legs off a donkey. If they're doing that, that's amazing. That's what you want. You want them chat and tell you their life story.

I was once taught that when it comes to telemarketing, you want to keep a potential client on the phone for as long as possible. Yet in our practices, if we are honest we most of the time want to get rid of people on the phone as quickly as possible. The goal is to form a relationship with them, like, "Hey, what's happening? How can I help?"

Then you need to track your stats. Keep a call log – "Mary's been called once, no answer; twice, no answer; third time, no answer, left message.

The reason its important to say track whether you left a message is so that you have continuity for your next call. e.g. "Hey, I left a message, did you get it?"

Before I tested this, I just assumed people knew it was us and they were trying to avoid us. But I tried calling from random numbers where they wouldn't know it was us and the results were the same.

So, the key to help you here is mix it up between mobile and landline. But the big key is when you use a mobile phone, do not leave a message. The reason is because if people get a missed call from a mobile number, they're much more likely to phone that number back and they do.

When you call from a landline, you can leave a message but mix it up between the two.

Next, be prepared to "date." You don't even get to a "No." It's like, "How can we help you? What more information can I send you?"

It's from one bridge to another bridge. When is your next health talk? Invite them to the next health talk. Is there a free taster session they can come to?

This works really well. That's what we do, "A lot of people are just like you. They're not quite sure who to use and often they just need more information. Maybe this might work for you – a free taster session. Come along and speak to one of our docs. There's no obligation. They're just going to tell you what's going on and it's completely free."

You can add to this, "The only thing you need to do is pay for x-rays but only if they are clinically required." Then offer them another bridge. So, keep offering bridges and be prepared to date.

Moving on from the Challenge of Free

Now, I just want to say a word here about one of the white elephants in the room. I know what you're thinking.

You probably don't like the words "free" or "free care."

Some people have told me, "Never give adjustments away for free." And I agree with that BUT there is most definitely a place for "free" in your practice.

So, let me tell you about a few studies.

There's a great book called Predictably Irrational. It covers a study where they took some chocolates – Hershey's Kisses and a Lindt truffle. The Hershey's kiss was one cent and the Lindt truffle was 26 cents. 40 percent of the people went for the kiss and 40 percent of the people went for truffle.

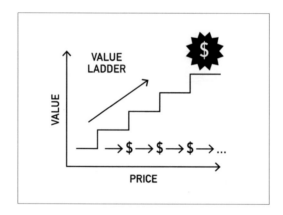

They repeated the study. They made the cheap one free and then dropped the price of the truffle by the same amount so that it was 25 cents. Ninety percent of the people went for the free option.

The price difference was the same as in the first study and yet now we have a 90 percent uptake. The message is when you offer something free, you drop the risk.

Then in the next part of the study, they made it minus 1 cent, which meant they gave you one cent if you took the Hershey kiss first and they dropped the Lindt truffle to 15 cents and it made no difference to the uptake compared to free.

The word free is irresistible... free reports, free discovery session, free health talk.

Everyone wants something free. It doesn't matter how much money you have.

So that's the first thing I want to say.

Secondly, I'm all about science of marketing so I want to introduce you to something called a "Value Ladder."

A value ladder is what someone progressively spends with you over time. They start with something free and then they go up.

A regular customer funnel often looks like the following.

You have a lead magnet which is free, then you have a trip wire. An example of a "trip wire" is something like a free book where all you have to do pay for shipping.

The reason they get you to pay for the shipping is because it's a trip wire.

A regular customer funnel

1. Lead magnet (free)
2. Trip wire (people show commitment 2 ways)
3. Core service
4. Upsells, cross-sells, profit maximizers
5. Return paths
6. Referrals

If they can get you to pay $2.99 for shipping, your percentage chance of becoming a buyer goes up about 80 percent.

Then you have core service up-sells, down-sells, cross-sells. Then you have return path and then you have referrals. This is a general model and is not specific to chiropractors.

When you look at dentists, they have a phenomenal value ladder. You can start with free teeth cleaning and you can end up with cosmetic dentistry worth $20,000 and more.

So, they get free teeth cleaning and then they pay for the teeth whitening and for braces. So, it starts out free, then it's like $30, then it's like $150, $1,000 and then it's like $10,000 and up.

This is from a book by Russell Brunson called Dotcom Secrets. What's so interesting about this book is one of his best friends is a chiropractor. So, he actually mentions chiropractors in the book and says chiropractors have got a tough time because we don't have a great value ladder. We don't often have something low priced or introductory before the adjustment and traditionally we don't have much of an "upsell" other than the adjustment.

Yes, you've got retention, but there's no product or major service at a much higher value. Now, I'm not into products. I hate products. In fact, there's almost no products in my business. I'm just not a product guy so it doesn't excite me so I'm not going to ask you to create products and stuff like that.

I'm just saying you need to be aware of the fact that in our industry we have to be OK with sometimes giving free stuff away.

Many say you should never give the adjustment away for free and I agree in 95% of the cases. I do however break the rule once or twice a year.

For example, at Christmas, a big campaign for reactivations where someone hasn't been in for three or six months and they've spent a substantial amount of money with us. I'll be like, "Come back, new year, new you – the adjustment is on us. We'd love to see you."

One coach who teaches not to give adjustments for free, he's a good friend of mine and he came and spent some time with me and looked at the results of my marketing campaign and said, "Wow dude, how did you get such great results?"

So, I told him I was giving away free adjustments and he said, "Dude, I do that all the time."

The reason I hadn't done it before was because of him. So, I realised that these guys who preach that you shouldn't give free adjustments away are giving free adjustments away all the time .

However, I literally break that rule at maximum twice a year. Otherwise, it's something else, it's a free consultation, a free report, a free talk, free something and maybe twice a year I'll break rule.

Trust me, it works very well.

PART TWO

THE NEW PATIENT AVALANCHE BLUEPRINT

THE NEW PATIENT AVALANCHE BLUEPRINT

In this part, I'm going to share with you the exact steps that I followed to grow to eight offices, attract more than 10,000 new patients a year and earn over $7 million revenue.

Here are the components:

1. Make More of Screenings

2. Maximize Results from Talks/Events

3. Harness the Full Power of Email

4. Take Advantage of Print and Other Media

5. Make the Best of Facebook

6. Leverage Your Existing Clients

7. Profit from Holiday Campaigns

Honestly, that's a $7 million blueprint right there.

In this chapter, we'll go through them all in detail but let's start with an overview of some of these elements.

Screenings

With screenings, you've got your community events and then you've got corporate events. I'll also talk about how you can do screenings successfully without you even being there. That's really screening in a nutshell. I know it's not sexy but it works.

Talks and Events

With talks and events, you've got outside the clinic, meaning going to schools and businesses etc – again community and corporate, sometimes they are correlated with the screening. I'm going to cover that.

—Surgery cheese + wine ?? meet the chiro host

Then you've got talks done inside the clinic for potential clients that have never been to see you before but have opted in for a free informational talk very similar to a "dinner with the Doc" event. I'm going to teach you how to do this. This is very powerful.

I have said that if I had to start all over again in a practice in a clinic by myself, I would throw so much money at this it's unbelievable. This has to be marketing nirvana if you can pull it off regularly. Imagine your adjusting and you come to the end of your shift and while you've been doing that your team have been greeting all the attendees (sometimes as many as 50) and you simply walk in, deliver a killer informational talk and you get 50-80% of them to purchase a new patient examination right there. They get to know you. They get to see your clinic and you get to offer them something in your environment.

I just think it's the greatest marketing source of all time. It does take more work than say just a one touch campaign on Facebook, but it is worth it.

Then you've got talks for your practice members, where you've got your orientation classes, etc. It's hard to measure return on investment, but I can assure you that not only will it increase your retention but it will undoubtedly also get you new patients as you new patients attending these "orientation" classes are encouraged to bring family and friends.

Facebook

Clearly there are other options such as Instagram and Snapchat but for now I'm all in on Facebook. There is going to be a time when too many people are using Facebook and the cost per lead is going to go through the roof because that's exactly what happened with Google.

We do need to learn about other things but leave that to me and let me teach you. You can't do everything, so focus on Facebook right now because that's your biggest return on investment. We've already talked about some of the things you can do on Facebook and we'll go through it in more detail shortly.

Referrals and Holiday Campaigns

This is a big one. Now, you might have noticed that in my blueprint I hadn't mentioned reactivation, internal referrals, etc. That's because, for me, I lump that into this section. A holiday campaign essentially has a referral part to it. "For Easter, it's vital to get the whole family checked." That's a referral campaign.

Then they've also got a reactivation section. For example for our Easter campaign we went through, who we are targeting, what our offer is, how we are structuring the emails. Are we texting them. Are we sending them a voice message by a text? We will teach you this.

Then you've got a new clients campaign that is around the theme your marketing (Easter, Halloween etc).

Sometimes you'll also do a holiday campaign that's just for goodwill. For instance, it's the only time we ever do this. We don't serve coffee or give out unhealthy treats like chocolates etc in our clinics. We serves herbal teas and things like that. But for easter and other holiday campaign we will sometimes offer branded "treats" etc.

They are branded chocolates, so each chocolate has a wrapper on it. Inside the wrapper is a surprise gift worth $160, which is a free initial consultation for a family member or something. We give thousands of these out. So that's just a goodwill campaign and do we see a return investment on that. I don't measure it massively.

Making the Campaign Successful

In each of those campaigns, there are different elements, skills and media that make it successful. The actual campaign is not really the thing. It's getting to a point of being good enough at the media in each of those where you're going to find your biggest traction.

Is good enough, good enough? I promise you now that perfectionism is the absolute killer of dreams. I want you to all be ok with being good enough. The stupidest thing I've ever heard in my entire life was someone saying, "If you cant do something properly, don't do it at all", that is absolutely not true. Sometimes good enough, is good enough.

I promise you now that perfectionism is the absolute killer of dreams.

———

There was a great story I heard Dan Kennedy tell. I've been a big Dan Kennedy fan for years and been a member of his inner circle group for a long time. He once told a story about when they used to get orders, his accountant was in charge of sending the boxes out for a while when they got an order for information products.

He was looking for his accountant and he was never around. When he caught up with him, he asked, "What are you doing all day?" and he said, "Well, I'm busy doing the wrapping of the boxes."

Dan said, "Bring me a box" and it was the most beautifully packed box that he's ever seen. He said, "Stop that right now. I want you to take 10 seconds to put a piece of tape on it and send it out." Good enough is good enough.

Sometimes, sending an email, I don't care how bad it is, is better than sending nothing. Good enough is often good enough.

There's an old saying, if you're not incredibly embarrassed by your first launch, email campaign, reactivation campaign, screening or talk, when you look back, then you haven't gone fast enough.

If you're not incredibly embarrassed by the first set of emails you've sent, you haven't gone fast enough. I know you want that email to look perfect, but trust me just send it out.

You'll just make more money, serve more people and make a bigger impact every time you do it. That's all that happens.

I remember I went to a big marketing conference a few years ago in America, and there was a young guy and his rental in New York city for his martial arts studio was a hundred grand a month. A multi-million-dollar martial arts studio for goodness sake, and he was prepared to take on that risk.

He was a young guy and and he had recently started using video advertising on his website etc when it wasn't the norm. I remember asking him is he used a professional film crew to do it and I will never forget what he said. He was like, "No, I just hold up a camcorder." And I was like, "But isn't it a bit messy?"

He said these lines to me which I'll never forget, "Whatever I put up there, no matter how messy, is better than what I currently have up there, which is nothing."

It's not the "thing" it's the media making up the thing that matters...

Need to be GOOD ENOUGH at:
- Basics of copywriting
- Basics of email marketing
- Basics of phone or telemarketing
- Basics of direct mail
- Basics of what to put in newsletter
- Basic talk structure
- Basics of "platform" selling
- Basics on Facebook
- Basics of Text marketing

So, this is your job. Throw lots of stuff on the wall and, whatever sticks, you go with. Most of us don't test nearly enough stuff.

Embrace sloppy success because that is where the power is. You will learn way more from a mistake than you will from a success. Your job is to make as many mistakes as quickly as possible. When in doubt, take action.

My job is to help you get good enough at copywriting, basic email marketing, basic phone marketing, telemarketing, basic direct mail, basics to putting out a newsletter, the basic talk structure, the basics of platform selling… that's converting someone from a talk into a client… basics of Facebook and the basics of text marketing.

STEP #1: MAKE MORE OF SCREENINGS

I have to start here with an unsexy banker alert! Earlier I asked if you were you ok with an unsexy business that serves more people and makes more money with more time and less stress – and this is unsexy!

We're talking about screenings and we're talking about one of the lowest costs per lead and one of the most consistent sources of new clients that has literally built my business in the beginning. It can also be structured so that it's virtually passive, meaning you don't even have to be there.

I'm absolutely convinced that as you go through this book, you'll say to yourself several times, "I know that" or "I've forgotten that."

But remember I said that you get bored of your bankers. I get bored with them, everyone gets bored of their bankers. But imagine you told any business on the planet that they could make several million dollars from a specific source of new customers and they chose not to it, because they were too lazy or too bored of it. You would think they are crazy. In essence we kinda do that all the time in most of our practices at some point.

Here's the thing, it's the single most underestimated form of new client lead generation.

It's one of the easiest bankers you could possibly do. I know that everyone's more interested in the sexy Facebook stuff but this is just a huge source of new clients for us. We do so well from it.

It requires very little skill, it's simple, but it's not easy. It requires unprecedented levels of "no ego".

I often ask myself, "Why don't more people do this?" but I'm convinced it's because ego takes us out of the game.

We all know it's not glamorous. We've all done it before, but the challenge with it is to consistently do it. I'm going to teach you how to consistently do it.

I love that this is not easy.

Screenings

- The single most underestimated form of new client generation...
- One of the easiest "bankers"
- Requires VERY LITTLE SKILL and
- It is so simple... but not easy...
- Requires unprecidented levels of "no ego"
- The secret to success... Just show up

It's probably not a great example now, but, the famous cyclist Lance Armstrong, who won the Tour de France multiple times, said in his book that when he woke up in the morning and it was pouring with rain and it was miserable, he used to love it because he knew that it was hard.

He loved that it was hard because he knew that he was stronger than everyone else mentally.

He was like, "the harder the better, because I just know I'm mentally stronger than them."

So, I love that this is simple but I also love that it's not easy! If you just stick to the process I'm going to teach you, you have just paid for this book 1000 times over, by implementing some of the stuff just on this one chapter.

Screening – Definition and Benefits

The definition of the screening is an "inside or outside event where you set up a 'stall' and you offer passer-by trade an opportunity to get a posture check or spinal check/ assessment.

The prospect is then offered an opportunity to come into the office for an initial examination at a substantially reduced fee that they pay at the event to secure their spot."

That's all a screening is. You offer them an opportunity to come in.

Types of screenings... I'm going to go through this later in more detail.

You have fairs and fetes. These are the best. Get a CA to look for every possible fair and fete coming up in the summer that you could possibly find and go to every single one.

Screening – Definition

- Inside or outside event where you set up a "stall" and offer passer-by trade an oppportunity to get an "posture check" or "spinal check/assessment."
- The prospect is then offered an opportunity to come into the office for an initial examination at a substantially reduced fee that they pay at the event to secure their spot.

The beautiful thing about them is they're so cheap. But they are also brilliant.

Now they're hard to find because you'll see them on lamp posts and things like that, but you have to tell everyone on your team that this is important.

Then shopping malls. They will often make you book a week at a time, so it can be labour-intensive to pull it off, but I'll teach you how to do that in a moment.

For supermarkets, we use a third party to book them, so you just book it through them.

It's always best to go through the local manager because often they'll say to do it for free or they'll just charge you on the side. The only problem in any of those industries is the managers change rapidly, so you lose your contact. That's why we often need to book it through a third party that specialises in this type of marketing event.

Local stores are great. They're usually free. I have someone on my team who has done an awesome job of just putting in the effort to build the relationships and we get into local stores and local health shop or whatever.

Types of screenings

- Fairs and fetes (low cost)
- Shopping malls.
  - Often have to do a week, labour intensive but still great
- Supermarket
- Local stores (great + free)
- Ninja move - gyms (1–5)
  - Pop in weekly for 2 hours in evening
- Corporate

Go spend two hours. Some people go, "I only got three clients." You only got three clients, but your lifetime value is $1,000 and you've got a 60 percent conversion rate. So, you just made yourself $2,000 in two hours.

Ninja move alert – gyms. I love gyms. I've worked with hundreds of associates and it's still a fact that if they show up to the screenings, they are more successful than there colleagues.

Corporate events are amazing. I'd go as far as to say corporates are pretty close to being the best. But how do you get in? I'm going to tackle that in a different segment because it's that important. Corporates are amazing.

Advantages and Disadvantages

The advantage of screening is it just works. Don't think too much about it. They are simple to do, many venues to choose from. You get payment before they come in on the day, which is awesome. You create rapport before they even come in, if you're the person actually doing them, then your conversions of theses clients into care are ofte really great.

The ninja move with screenings is that they can be done without you. I'm going to show you how to do this.

The best in the profession still do them in some way shape or form, even if they don't like to readily admit it. Trust me.

Advantages

- It just works, don't think too much
- Simple to do
- Many venues to choose from
- You get payment before they come in for day
- Create rapport before they come in
- Therefore. better conversions
- Ninja move... can be done without you
- Best in the profession still do it
- Very low cost per client

So, success leaves clues. I agree, it's not glamorous to do screenings, but these guys still do them.

Disadvantages

- Time consuming
- Cost involved - venue, equipment, staff
- Not glamorous
- Fatigue (hard to be consistent)
- Access to venues changes due to staff turnover or policy changes internally

Screenings have a very low cost per client, specifically if you are the person at the screening.

Disadvantages are that they are time-consuming and sometimes the cost involved can climb quickly.

Obviously, there's a cost involved such as the venue, the equipment and staffing the venue, which I highly recommend you do.

It's not glamorous. You need no ego to be able to do this. Fatigue, it's hard to be consistent.

In my list earlier of core reasons why practices fail to market themselves, one of the most important is lack of consistency. For this, you know it works and you are probably really good at it.

Someone I was working with for a while eventually went and did a bit of screening after not doing one for 15 years and he got over 60 new patients in an afternoon.

Just think about what that is worth to him. If you've got 50 percent conversion and your lifetime value is $1,000, you're talking about $30,000 for just showing up to a screening.

However, I'm telling you it's not about the screening you do and get 60 people, it's about the 40 screenings you do and get five at each.

That is where it's at. It's the showing up to one a week and getting five and being ok with it and making sure your cost per lead is low.

Screenings — What You Need

So, what do you need? You need:

- A venue
- A process on the day
- After the event follow-up, which is very important

We've already talked about the different types of venue so let's talk more about what you need to do on the day.

One the following page is the checklist we use in my business.

I'm not going to go through it in detail. It's all there.

Then supplies, you need a SAM machine, you need scales, you need a table, you need a skirt for the table, you need a spine model and a degeneration model. You need some way for people to pay.

If you don't want to go to the investment yet of buying a SAM machine, what I'd recommend is you can buy a pull up that has a grid and you can just buy the scales which are the same scales that are used in the SAM machine. They are like $30.

Get it up there and you can start there. Then allocate your profits from that to investing in a SAM machine.

I'm telling you now, we always like to get 100 new clients before we open a practice. We've always done that through screenings.

CHECKLIST

Before leaving for the screening – check you have the following:

- SAM Machine and top U-Shaped part that fits onto the poles (in bag)
- Poles (In pole bag)
- Roller banner – 1 MINIMUM per gig (in bag)
- Table
- Table skirt (usually in the box with spine)
- Spine and stand
- Wheelie bag

Wheelie bag contents:

- Strings for SAM Machine
  (Green – 1 x Long, 3 x Short. Red – 1 x Long, 3 x Short)
- Orange Vouchers (x30)
- Booking forms (x30)
- Control Sheets (x10)
- Clipboards (x2)
- Credit card machine, cable and plug (in padded zip bag)
- Stapler
- Staples
- Till roll (x2)
- Pens
- Public Liability Insurance laminated sheet

For OUTDOOR events:

- Green Gazebo (in bag)
- Green sand weights (x4)
- Wooden platform base. Needed on grass. (1 x large rectangle for SAM machine to sit on and 2 shorter pieces to use to level under large board if needed)

Screenings – On the Day

Let's take a look at what you do on the day. I'm going to introduce you to the simplest screening process and script of all time.

It's important for it to be simple because if you hire associates, you can teach them a script until they're blue in the face and I'll guarantee that if you go into the exam room and you observe them, you'll find they're doing their own thing. It doesn't matter how hard you try to script them, they don't do it if its not simplified.

The problem with all the scripts out there is that there are many people teaching good scripts, but they're not taking into consideration that there is a different motivation between owners and associates.

There's a different motivation level between when you put a script in front of an associate and make them do it as opposed to when you do it and you have to pay the bills.

I've worked with more associates than just about anyone on the planet and I will tell you, I don't care what you do, they are not doing the scripts that you tell them to do. What I've learned is what is the least amount that they need to master to be efficient? It's five simple steps.

So, this is what I've done with my screening scripts, because I've got a team doing it. What's the least they need to be doing to get a good enough result?

Here's the script.

Step #1: Get attention and get them to agree to the screening

There are so many ways to get attention. I'm going to give you an example in a moment, but just a heads up, nobody knows what a screening is. So, don't ask them if they want a screening.

I'm going to teach you a little cool line that has been shown to increase people stopping from 29 percent to 70 percent.

Step #2: Get them to complete the questionnaire

Then, once they agree to the screening, they need to fill out the questionnaire first.

There are many variations of the questionnaire. I'm not saying that ours is perfect, but it's certainly good enough.

The optimum thing about it is you have to know their "pain". If you don't know the pain, it's very difficult to do the screening and you need to know this before they jump on the screening machine.

So, let them fill out the form. A reason we use to justify this is that we need consent.

Once they fill out the form, you take the form from them and you need to scan the form. Just to put yourself at a point of awareness, you need to know what's going on with them before they get on the machine.

Step #3: Do the screening

There are different ways you could do screenings, but all qualified chiropractors know how to assess someone's posture.

When you're doing that, make sure that you've got your analogies. Analogies are stories that sell, really stories sell. That's like, "Extra two pounds down one side, that's like two bags of sugar. Imagine walking around with that all down one side all day.

Analogies are very important. So, we train our screeners on those analogies.

With this screening, I'm going to say that your job is not to answer every one of their questions. Our screeners will often tell me to please not let the doctor come. They don't want the chiropractor there sometimes.

They sell less with the chiropractor there because we are so intent on trying to solve the problem that we speak too much, and we out-speak them into not taking the deal.

My business partner is probably one of the best screeners I've ever seen. He doesn't even put them on the SAM machine. He just says, "It's a great deal. $30 instead of $100." He never puts them on the machine.

Now I would recommend putting them on the SAM machine and you do your posture assessment. This is where the key happens.

Step #4: Link posture to pain

When you get them off the posture machine, the next part, the setup, you need to just link their posture to some of the things you found on their questionnaire.

So, this is all done by a very simple question, **"Can you see how your … … can be contributing to your … …?"**

For example, "Can you see how the extra weight down your left-hand side can be contributing to the pain you're getting down the left-hand side?"

So, you've got to link their posture to their pain. And it's important to get a yes.

Step #4: Test close

Once you get a 'yes', that's called a test close. Once you get a 'yes', here's the next most important question you'll ever learn from me, **"How important is it for you to … …?"**

You've got to fill in what you feel comfortable saying here. "Listen John, can you see how this can be contributing to your lower-back pain?" Yes. "How important is it for you to get this fixed?"

I know working in chiropractic, some of you are going to feel uncomfortable with the word 'fixed', but it's a powerful word or 'sorted'. Because the body heals itself. I get that.

But whatever you feel comfortable with, use that "How important is it for you to get this properly looked at?"

It's got to sit well with you. Otherwise, you're just going to look like a bulldog chewing on a wasp when you say it.

By the way, can you use that sentence in your Report of Findings also.. It's the best sentence ever.

Step #5: Close

Once you've got the "very," then you just do the close. Remember, selling is a process of subconsciously getting people down a process of yeses or micro-commitments.

"Can you see how this has contributed to that?" Yes. "How important is it for you to get this sorted?" Very. "Awesome, I can help you." It's really easy. It's a conversation.

I want to run through the close a little bit more. When they say "very," you're going to say, "Great, we can really help you. We're actually here at (wherever it is) as part of our community outreach. Although today was insightful, I don't want to guess with your health. So, let's get you properly looked at. Normally an initial consultation is (whatever it is). But, because we are here today in partnership with (whoever), it's just $50."

There is also an important line once you say the price difference.

So, if you go, "Because we're here today, it's just $20 or $30 instead of..." you want to say, **"Much better, right?"**

It's important to get a "yes" here.

This is really high-level stuff in sales and marketing. It's impossible to say, "No, it's not better" because it is better.

All of you have been to big speaking events where they sell from the stage. Now that I've taught you the secrets, you'll see them all do it. Every great trainer from stage does this.

The next thing you say is, "All we need to do today is get you sorted with your payment and a time to come in." You want to book the appointment right there.

If you have cloud-based booking systems, it is so worth the extra to get them booked into that or simply do it old school with a pen and paper on a spreadsheet showing available slots.

Remember, if you let them walk away, you can expect to make at least 10 phone calls before you get hold of them. That is an exhausting thought so do your best to book them right there and then.

This was my $350,000 mistake, that's the minimum I lost because of that.

Assumption one was I thought that I could just call them. But I looked at my stats and was getting them one every 10 calls. So, we were just drowning in leads.

Assumption two, was I thought that if they had paid for the voucher, surely they'd come along. But they don't. So, I lost 1,500 new patients because of that one mistake.

So, do not let them walk away. Get them booked them in the diary right there. That was my mistake, don't make the same mistake I made.

Ninja Move – Upsell

Now, a ninja move. This is what nobody's doing, and it changes your stats dramatically. It's the upsell.

A billion-dollar business was built on this concept. You may be familiar with this line, "Would you like fries with that?"

When you offer them another opportunity to buy, 33 percent will say "Yes."

A billion-dollar industry was built on that sentence because 33 percent of people just say yes. If you then ask, "Would you like a soft drink as well?" another 33 percent of people say yes to that because they are in the buying cycle.

So, when you offer them another opportunity to buy, 33 percent will say "yes." So, this is the friends and family deal.

Once someone has bought a $30 voucher, you would just simply say to them, "Would you like to get another one for any of your friends and family?" You could offer that for $10 or $15.

Our stats show similar results, one in four, say "yes" to the upsell.

So, this changes your stats dramatically. If you are doing even 12 screenings a year, and every third or fourth person says yes to an upsell, you're going to change your stats big time. So always ask for an upsell.

You've got two formats of a screening:

- One-person format – one person is doing the whole screening

- Two-people format – two people are involved. One acts as the attention grabber and another as screener, probably the doc, then hand back to the first person to do the booking.

If it's one-person format, you're doing both and it's very cost efficient, but sometimes it's harder to maintain energy than with the other structure.

With the two-person model, the attention grabber gets them to fill out a form and hands them over to the doc, who gets them to the point where they say, "How important is it for you to get this sorted."

When they answer "very" they hand them back to the grabber to close the deal and get them booked in.

Having two people is great for energy and works especially well for fairs and fetes and high-volume events where there's lots of people. You can even have more at very busy events.

The Secret of Pre-Suasion

I just want to quickly tell you about this from the book "Pre-Suasion" by Robert Cialdini, who also wrote the very famous book "Influence." I saw him live in San Diego and he taught me this.

Studies have found that if you stop people on the street asking them to fill out a questionnaire, about 29 percent of people will stop and agree to fill out the questionnaire.

However, if they ask one simple question before, the response rate jumps to 70 percent. The question was, "Would you consider yourself someone that is helpful?"

Now if I say yes and I don't help you fill out a questionnaire, there's a disconnect.

They did another study where they asked people to test a new soft drink in the street, and 27 percent of people agreed to try it and give feedback. When they asked one question first, which was, "Do you consider yourself someone that's adventurous and likes to try new things?" it would jump to over 70 percent.

So how does this relate to us? You could say something like:

- "Would you consider yourself someone who values their health?"
- "Would you say your health is really important to you?"

Who's going to say they don't value their health or that it isn't important to them? Then, once, they said yes, we go, "Great, then you're the sort of person that's really going to be interested in this."

It can be very powerful. So, try and work it into your scripts.

Biggest Mistakes

Here are some of the biggest mistakes people make with screenings.

One is to say, "Do you want a screening?" People don't know what a screening is. So that's a big mistake. You have to ask a question they can relate to.

Mistake number two, not getting symptoms before the screening. You've got to get the symptoms on the sheet before the screening. It's very important.

Next, not taking payment on the day. If you say, "Don't worry, you can pay when you come in," you'll get about a 90 percent no-show rate.

Biggest Mistakes

- "Do you want a screening?" They don't know what screening is, rather "When was the last time you had your spine checked? "or "Do you consider yourself someone who is health conscious?"
- Not getting symptoms before screening. Must get symptoms (Questionaire "for consent") before screening and link to problem found
- Not taking payment on the day (90% no-show rate if no pay)
- Not booking the appointment on the day at the screening... or pre-framing the call to get booked in.

We still do it from time to time, say if someone doesn't have their wallet on them in the gym, but then you must phone them straight away and get the payment, "I'm going to call you today to take the payment." Otherwise it's just a waste of time and you'll get a 90 percent no-show rate if you don't take payment on the day.

The other mistake is not booking the appointment on the day at the screening, or if you absolutely have to do it later pre-frame that they're going to get a call within the next few hours.

Achieving Consistency – Done Without You

The whole point to this whole conversation is how do you make this consistent?

Here's the thing. Very few practices are able to do this on a regular basis. But we do.

In the past, we've had anywhere from 5 to 10 a week. This is how we were able to get $7 million worth of revenue and up to 10 screenings a week – and I didn't go to a single one!

How did I do it? Hint – it has a lot to do with knowing what you can afford to spend on a client. That is the key to understanding how you make this work.

If you're not doing this, you're leaving thousands of dollars on the table.

You may not start this way. If you are starting a new clinic, get out there and do it yourself. Just get out in the community. Do it as often as you can. But you may want to do a combination of these to keep it consistent. The thing that you're missing is consistency.

Done Without You

- You may not start with this...
- The thing that you're missing to make this consistent...
- If you have a Team then they can share the load... need to set context from the word go.
- Be careful to rely on DC's
- Or a few part timers that do it for you... (my favourite)
- I would suggest a combination of the two...
- Meaning that if you have someone take responsibility to setup and pack down...
- You just show up and help...
- That will give you biggest ROI (time and finance)
- And most importantly give you a better chance at being CONSISTENT

If you have a team, then they can share the load. But if you're hiring associates and a team, then you want to set context before they start. You can set context before they start in your core values ... one of our core values in my team is that "we always show up".

It can be a challenge to get the team to do this consistently one tip is to also have a few part-timers that help you with this. I would suggest the combination of having your team do it and a few part-timers helping you, meaning that if you have someone taking responsibility for setting up and packing down, then you can just pop in.

That's the base. If you have someone responsible for being there and setting up, packing up, you still go, or your team still goes, but at least you are showing up. Just show up and help where you can.

This is going to be your biggest return on investment time-wise and most importantly, give you a chance to be consistent. So, this is very important.

This is another Ryan-ism – "it's not about showing up good, it's about showing up at all". All you have to do is simply out-show-up everyone else.

Next Steps

The plan going forward is you've got three options:

- Base level, which is one screening per month.

- Major league, where you're going to be doing two per month

- All-Star level, which is four per month.

So how much is that worth to you if you do one a month? Sometimes you can get between 20 and 30 a day, but let's say across the year you do 12 screens and get 10 at each, that's potentially 120 new clients.

This is why it's so important to know your lifetime value because everything comes back to it and your conversion rate is key.

Let's say your conversion rate is 50% to be conservative, so we're looking at 60 clients that you convert. If your lifetime value is $1,000, you could easily make yourself $60,000 just by doing one screening a month.

For most of you, that's like 60 percent, 70 percent profit. It makes a big difference.

If you have a high conversion, and a $2,000 lifetime value, which some of you have, you could make $120,000 extra for going to one screening a month.

I will teach you the bankers like this all day long over the sexy, shiny stuff that comes along on Facebook or whatever.

But I'm telling you right now, you can put an extra $100,000 in your bank account and help a lot more people just by doing some screenings.

STEP #2: MAXIMIZE RESULTS FROM TALKS AND EVENTS

This chapter is all about Talks, also known as "bums in seats." The only objective really is to get bums in seats in different environments.

Why Talks?

Here's the thing about talks… I've explored so many ways to generate leads in many different businesses but I'll never forget what one of my greatest coaches and mentors said to me at a point in my career where I was starting to get a little blasé.

I was starting to get good at online marketing and I wasn't so sure that I believed this statement when he said it to me at first, but I cant tell you just how true it is, he said, "Of all the ways to generate leads, there is still nothing that can replace the power of live events."

When you talk, you're automatically perceived as the expert.

I now know he was right. I don't care how good we get at generating new patients online, there is nothing that replaces the power of a live event. Nothing. All the fancy online tools cannot ever replace the ability to generate the amount of leads and the quality of leads from some type of talking environment in such a short period of time, provided you can find the opportunities to get in front of people.

It's just about getting bums in seats if you can set up a talk… and I understand that's a big fear for a lot of people, but I'll show you a few easy hacks around that so that you don't even have to talk at all with some of them.

There is still nothing on the planet that will beat the quality of lead and speed of lead from a live event. I mean, within 20 minutes you can stand in front of a thousand people and you can generate 500 leads.

Here's the thing, what do Ryan Deiss, Frank Kern and Russell Brunson have in common? If you don't know who they are, check them out. They are some of the biggest names on the planet in the online marketing space.

One thing they all have in common is that they are the biggest online marketers on the planet and they all STILL speak regularly onstage around the world. They leverage the power of live events.

It still amazes me to this day that these guys are doing many million's of dollar's online, yet they still get in a car, get on a plane, fly across the country and stand up and talk for free.

There is still nothing on the planet that will beat the quality of lead and speed of lead from a live event.

———————————

I was in the room with Frank Kern live in San Diego, he's one of my online marketing heroes. I think he's making about a million a month online at the moment. He stands up and writes his speaker fee on the board. A big zero.

So why did he go there and stand up in front of 700 people when he can make more money lying in his bed? It's a simple thing because there is still nothing that can beat the power of a live event. There's no substitute for gathering people together.

When you talk, you're automatically perceived as the expert and will naturally attract the clients that you want to work with. That's a big point.

Types of Talk

There are three main types of talks:

- Orientation classes, something you do regularly in your practice

- You talking to a company, similar to "lunch and learns".

- Talk in the clinic for external attendees, people who come to you and who want to learn from you.

So, which of those is the best? That's a little bit of a trick question.

As I've said before, successful people don't think 'either/or', they think 'and'. There's no best. They're all relevant.

Going to talk in company environments is amazing, there's so little resistance.

The advantage of number three is they literally come to you. How beautiful is that? You have 40 people or 20 people or 10 people rock up to your clinic. They come to you. You just finished your adjustments and they are waiting for you.

They're all fantastic in their own rights. So, you want to be thinking of these as three separate things. Even though I'm covering this in talks, this is how you leverage and scale your business straight away from this one chapter.

You've got three different areas that you can leverage straight away and that's how you get multiple quantum leaps in income.

Talk Type #1: Orientation Classes

I'm going to start by talking about the orientation class or health class within a practice. There are practices across the planet that literally rely solely on this to grow their practice. People bring a partner, a friend, it can be in the form of a dinner with a doc.

I have been involved with practices where we did this religiously and I've been involved in many, many practices where they don't do it at all. Without doubt, this will positively affect the retention in any business, not just a chiropractic business.

But, big warning, I've almost never seen this done effectively or consistently in a large multi doc practice, unless the owner in the clinic or one doc takes the lead role. I'll tell you why.

Your associates really struggle to see the value of this or rather they may simply really struggle with this as you're also asking them to partake in arguably one of the greatest fears, public speaking. If people are asked in a poll about their greatest fear, they will rate public speaking above death.

That means that, at a funeral, they would rather be in the box than say the eulogy. So, that's a big thing you're asking from your associates.

It can be done weekly or it can work fortnightly.

We're often taught that these talks are done to educate our clients and we're going to teach them exactly how we need them to be. But I'm telling you now, because I'm involved in so many other businesses, that's just not why we see the results.

When you look at the statistics across other businesses, their real effect comes from simply the gathering. It's not really what's said. It's going to the effort of the gathering... getting people in a room as a team and creating fellowship. That is where the likability factor comes through.

While a great talk and a great presenter makes a difference, it's much more about doing them in the first place as opposed to what's being said in them.

I don't care what anyone says about "educating" them etc., I'm telling you now that in the world of business that just doesn't add up.

I'm not saying there isn't an element of that that comes into it, but simply doing them religiously and putting people in the room and showing up, that's where you get the results.

So, the secret is actually just doing them consistently. But that's tough because you need the whole team to get involved behind that.

People do business with people and this massively increases the ability of getting your prospect to a point where they know, like and trust you. That's why we do it, is to get people to bond with you and your team.

But usually it's around a personality. That's why it's very difficult for it to work if you're not choosing one personality to wrap it all around, whether it's you as the practice owner, whether it's the one associate in the practice that's going to take these on board.

This massively increases the ability of getting your prospect to a point where they know, like and trust you.

———

I promise you that my business would not exist today if I did not do live events, it just would not exist. It's the effect of getting people into a room and gathering. It's the fellowship getting everyone in the room.

The biggest online guys in the world still get all the students in a room once a year, so there is absolutely no doubt in my mind that going to the extra effort of getting people in the room will massively improve your business.

And how I know is because I read all these business journals, and if you're familiar with Tupperware parties or other network marketing businesses, a few years ago those were huge across the world.

They built that whole industry on live events and, since the advent of online marketing, a few of the network model bosses thought it was a bit of a pain to get everyone together for meetings.

They were doing weekly meetings with five or six or 10 people in a room, doing a regional monthly meeting and then doing a slightly bigger quarterly meeting where they went to a hotel and they had all the costs of setting up the venue.

They actually decided as a group, as a company decision that they were getting rid of all their events and it almost put every one of those companies into bankruptcy. So, they quickly brought back those live events.

Going to the effort of putting people in the room and creating the fellowship is honestly where the magic happens. So, there is no substitute for a gathering. There never will be. They'll never ever be replaced. We will never get to a point where we don't meet live in person events.

Should you be doing them? There is no doubt. Sometimes what will happen is you're not quite sure whether this is really making a difference – should I really be doing this for three people?

I promise you, it makes a difference and every business should be using this strategy to increase new customers, retention and referrals.

So, the main point I wanted to leave you with is that doing them is better than not doing them without a shadow of a doubt no matter how amateurish or unpolished you may feel when you speak.

Talk Type #2: Corporate Events

Let's talk now about corporate events. This is when you're invited to speak or do screenings inside a corporate entity that has 20 plus employees. It is not desk assessments.

If I had a penny for every single time some other associate or someone I'm coaching says, "We've got to get in the desk assessment marketplace." I'm telling you now it's just not what you should be focusing on.

You want to become the invited guest as opposed to the unwanted pest.

In fact, it is a barrier to getting into companies. It's the reason you're not getting into companies if you're even saying you want to do a desk assessment.

You want to become the invited guest as opposed to the unwanted pest, and with that comes a huge amount of social proof and trust. That's why there's so little resistance when you get into these companies.

Without a doubt, it's the easiest "screening" you'll ever do in your life.

I've had many people do this for the first time, especially if they've done loads of screenings, and they'll almost always come to me and say something like, "It was like shooting fish in a barrel." Everyone just says, "It was the easiest sale I ever made in my life."

The hard work is getting in. But once you're in, just go to have fun because they are fantastic. You can get 30-100 new patients in a day.

If I had to start all over again, what I would do are the talks within the clinic and fill the room plus these corporate screenings.

So how do you get in? The inside track is always the best, meaning most of your clients in the clinic work somewhere. So, the simplest way to get into a company is ask your clients in the clinic.

You normally need a higher level of awareness from the team to do this because you shouldn't rely only on yourself. While that's possible, the level of awareness from the team to "pounce" on someone, when they see the history form is important. That's actually why on the history form you have a company name.

If all you did was make a one CA accountable to ask every single person who comes in, and they follow a script, you can build a list of companies.

I promise you this will generate some opportunities for you. So, you need to role play and train on this, so you get results and you just need to ask.

The best way to ask is simply to follow the script. "John, I notice that you work at XYZ... has anyone told you about our corporate health and wellbeing days?"

That's a term they may be familiar with because they often have to go to them. Or you could say, "Our free corporate lunch and learns." You want to say the word corporate in there and "free". You want to act as if this is something you do all the time.

Corporate lunch and learn. It's exactly what it says on the tin. If they say, "No, I haven't been told about them" the next part is very important.

The only thing you're trying to get from this conversation is a name of the best person to talk to. Now they might say something like, "I'm going to ask HR to give you a call." But you've just got to try. Just ask the question.

It doesn't matter if you don't get the answer, but you've got to ask the question, who is HR? What's her name? Even if it's the wrong person, you've got to get a name.

The only goal is to get a contact name and then I'm jumping ahead of myself, but when you phone that company, you also want to mention the client's name – if you have permission.

Simply say, "If I contact the company, can I mention that you passed on my details?" You just want to cover yourself for patient confidentiality and so on.

If you phone and say, "John Smith gave me your contact details and he asked me to call you and he said you might be expecting my call," nine times out of 10 they wouldn't have said anything about you, but at least you've got in.

We have generated over $2 million in the last five years just from this one source of leads.

Now the other way you get into companies is outbound, meaning that you phone them.

We do this full time and very aggressively. Meaning that we actually phone companies, we offer them opportunities for us to come into their business and offer a service.

This requires a lot of tenacity. When I tell people about our marketing, some people don't really want to hear all this stuff I'm telling you. They only want to know the easy way to get lots of new patients.

In the very first chapter, it was very clear to you guys that unfortunately there isn't an easy way. This takes tenacity. I know for a fact we phone companies 30, 40, 50 times before we get in sometimes.

Now, you don't have to be doing it as aggressively as we do it, but it's just the reality of the situation.

We have generated over $2 million in the last five years just from this one source of leads.

I've got 63 people in one 30-minute talk and we didn't even do screening.

Finding People to Call

How do you get the details of people to call for outbound calling? The single most important thing is you need a name, which I've mentioned. That's all you need.

I'm not saying don't phone a company without a name because there are sneaky ways to get in, but the goal is to get a name. You just want to be able to pick up the phone and say, "Hi, can I please speak to Mary Smith?"

Sometimes any name will do. Even if it's not the appropriate person, any name at the company will do sometimes.

For outbound research, we look at companies within a five-mile radius. You can definitely go for more than that because, even though the company's 10 miles away, you know that a lot of those employees are going to be living closer to your practice. So, you can definitely go further, but five miles is the best. You need the HR contact if possible.

To get HR contact details, there are many third party companies that will sell you these details. They will literally give you a list of HR people within five miles for as little as $200 to $300.

We gain a lot of traction from LinkedIn also. You get a free version and a paid one. You can search straight away for people who work in companies within a certain distance. Certainly, you can find your way around that very quick.

So, LinkedIn is big and then simply Googling companies is another source.

Successful people are always willing to do what unsuccessful people aren't.

Phoning people isn't easy, so I would go as far as incentivizing the team. Allowing for the cost of buying a list, there is no other cost. So, I would just say to someone on your team, "I'll pay you $200 or more every time we get into a company."

The only cost of the entire day is paying a person to book the gig.

These are the ones that I'd actually say you might want to go to yourself because they are so valuable, so simple. This does take courage, but it's so worth it.

Successful people are always willing to do what unsuccessful people aren't.

I was in San Diego and I had the privilege of hearing Daymond John speak. He's on Shark Tank and is the founder of FUBU.

He got asked a question, "What was a thing that you did in your early career that made the biggest impact?" He said, "I was broke. I had made mistakes. But I made a decision and it literally has changed my life. I made a decision to make 50 calls a day, no matter what. I didn't even know who I was going to call, but I made 50 calls, whether that was just to a new supplier, or whether it was to someone I needed to reach out to and ask for help."

Obviously, you don't need to take it to that extreme but what if you made five calls per day, every single day?

If you make five calls a day to companies, over a period of a year or two, you will trace back six figures to that guaranteed.

I said from the beginning you might find one or two techniques here and if you roll with them and rinse and repeat and scale, you are going to transform your practice.

Contacting Companies

When you phone a company, they may have a no-name policy, meaning when you say, "Who's the HR person in charge of xyz?" they won't tell you the name. That's why you need to phone with a name if you can. It's much better to say, "Can I speak to Kelly Smith in HR?"

You get this from your research. When you identify a company name, you want to get the name of the contact person in HR.

A sneaky little trick is if you have the name, you can say, "Before you put me through to Kelly, I was told that she was the right person to speak to with regards to health and well-being days. Is that correct?"

Then sometimes they'll say, "Actually, no, it's not Kelly, it's Mary." You can say, "Well I don't want to waste Kelly's time. Is it ok if I speak to Mary instead?"

Then you want to say something along the lines of, "It's about an upcoming health and wellbeing day."

Make sure you write all these names down, including the secretary's name who answers the phone, so you may need to ask her name. This is prospecting 101 but nobody teaches us.

If you don't get through, make a note to call back in a week, two weeks, a month. Then you pick up the phone and you say, "Hey Sarah, can I please speak to Mary Peters?"

So, you really want to leverage the name. It's all about the name. Then you need to follow a script.

We have a specific script that we use in my company and we follow it word for word. It's just a different level of competency when you call instead of thinking, "what do I say?"

We also have basic email templates that we use to make follow up easy.

When you find these companies, you've got to put yourself in their shoes. What's the biggest objection that we find when we go into companies? It's usually about money.

That's why you should not say you are offering desk assessments. Because they'll say, "I know what's going to happen. You're going to come in and say our desks are all bad and that we have to replace everything. We'll need new computers for 700 people and that's going to cost us $1 million. There's no way I want you in my business." So, you do not want to do that.

You need to tell them quickly that's not what you do.

Your job is simply to reassure them at that point and the script goes along the lines of, "Look, even if you had the best desk on the planet, we as chiropractors work with the functioning of the body. We help people get better without use of drugs and surgeries."

Tracking

Now, if there's one thing that you have learned from me it's that the fortune is in the follow up, so you've got to track this stuff.

There are fancy CRM systems you can use and all of that, but a simple spreadsheet will get you going.

It lists the names of the contact and when you're going to call them back.

You can give this to a person in your company to do and you just want to keep track of this.

We also have a comments section in there so that we can keep track of what they say on particular dates. Then when you phone back, you've got that information.

The Fish Bowl Trick

Here's a ninja move which if you implement this today, there's a chance you could be in a company in a few days. It's called the Fish Bowl promotion and it's simply have a big fish bowl at the front desk. It's a promotion to get company names and HR contact details.

You're going to tell people that they stand a chance to win a big prize – and it has to be a big prize like an iPad or a holiday for two.

Remember I got 60 clients from one event. Just work out what that is worth to you. It's crazy. We could possibly be talking about it being worth six figures to get into one company. So, is it worth paying for a holiday for two? I think you know the answer to that.

I know this sounds crazy, but there are companies that do this, and it's not as expensive as you think it is. So, don't be cheap with this.

You have to do this at least once a year and you need your team behind you. When we look back at the statistics and wonder if it was worth doing, you might say, "We didn't get into all that many companies … maybe six or seven." But the number of new clients we got from those seven companies was huge.

We actually did this, and we sent one of our clients on a holiday for two and it was awesome. It was worth tens of thousands of dollars for us.

All you need is a form at the front desk telling them how they can enter and some photos of the prize.

It simply has their name, email address, contact number, company name, name of HR best point of contact and contact number and the approximate number of employees. So, they have to fill that all out to enter.

By the way, this is the only time you are allowed to use a flyer!

Talk Type #3: Talks in Your Clinic for External Attendees

Our next segment is talks in your clinic for external attendees. I love these talks. I sometimes get frustrated because I think if we just had bigger audience sizes, we could do this so well.

However, the reality is we've only got a limited amount of people around our clinics, so this is not something that you can do all the time.

There are four elements to this:

1. Get people to register – i.e. bums in seats. We do this primarily from Facebook, which we'll talk about more in a later chapter.

2. Getting them to show up – this is very important. Do not assume that once they register, they're going to show up. I'm going to show you how to have a higher chance of them coming into the clinic and also how to warm them up, so they are more likely to buy when they come in.

3. Give them value on the day.

4. Convert attendees into clients.

Step #1: Getting People to Register

Although we'll talk about traffic sources later, I want to start by emphasising the importance of giving your talk a very appealing title.

When I really started looking at this world of driving people from online sources into the clinics, I was so excited. I couldn't wait to get people into talks about "Living Your Healthiest Life" and other wellness topics. I was so excited about the opportunity to educate our surrounding areas about what we do in vitalistic chiropractic.

I was going to cover topics such as "7 Essentials to Living Longer," "Five Keys to Being Your Healthiest," and "Pregnancy and Chiropractic." BUT nobody registered.

It was pretty heart-breaking for me. I was excited about getting people in the room who wanted to hear about how to live your healthiest life or how to be more successful as far as your health goes. I was so excited to talk about chiropractic, but nobody wanted to come.

This goes back to what I taught in chapter one – pain is the doorway to wellness care.

If you look at the billion-dollar industries on this planet, no-one does it better than the weight loss industry. They are not advertising how to be healthy, fit and good looking. They are first show you the photo of the sick person who may be obese or diabetic and how that person lost weight, but they start with the pain. They always start with the pain, the problem, and then agitate that.

I've previously talked about the copywriting formula – Problem, Agitate, Solve. And we've got another way of looking at it, it doesn't matter what marketing source you're talking about, and I don't even like saying it, but it's the truth and it's, "hurt them and heal them." Because no one takes action when you don't identify the problem first.

What we're trying to do is sell people on wellness and it's very difficult. Because people only take action when it's too painful to just stay where they are. The reality is we love our comfort zones and it's human nature to only take action when it's too painful to stay where you are.

So, give them what they want, then you can educate them as to what they can have over time. That is the miracle of chiropractic. As I mentioned before, B J Palmer himself said "Symptoms Sell."

I also said before that the customer is the hero, we are just the guide. And as badly as I want to fill a room with 20-50 people who want to be there to remove subluxation or restore the arc of life, it just doesn't work. You can't get people in the room.

So, we've got to sell people what they want, which in this case might be to get them out of excruciating pain. Then we can teach them what they can have later. The customer is the hero.

What we have found is that there are certain tested topics than that we use that work very well and others that haven't worked at all.

Here are some that didn't work:

- "Why resolutions don't work: The Power of Habits"

- "Getting the Best Out of Breastfeeding Workshop"

- "Surprising Benefits of Therapeutic Massage"

Here's the thing. If you look at all those subject lines of those talks, they don't really talk to a disease process. So, I'm just going to try to shift your mind. I guess our learning from it is that's it's not so much just even talking about a problem. It's about addressing some type of medical issue.

I know this is opposite to what we focused on in chiropractic, which is that we don't treat disease and we don't do those types of things and we have to be careful about saying we can cure things.

However, you can see the difference when I give you some examples of the highest response rates for topics we've done. For example, "Manage Back Pain and Sciatica Safely and Effectively."

Examples of this include:

- "Manage **Back Pain** and **Sciatica** Safely and Effectively"

- "How to manage **Chronic Fatigue Syndrome!**"

- "How to manage **Fibromyalgia** safely & effectively!"

- "Safe and Effective Ways to Manage the symptoms of **Autism**"

- "Managing the symptoms of **ADHD and Dyslexia** effectively"

- "How Manage **Arthritis** Effectively & Naturally!"

Now, let's be clear, we're not advertising that we can cure or heal these problems. We are advertising how to manage symptoms such as chronic fatigue syndrome.

The fact is, you don't even need to talk chiropractic in the beginning. You can talk about eating healthy and stretching and things like that. Then, you just educate people about chiropractic and with the right close, it's impossible for people to say no.

The best performing of these titles were the last three.

The one on managing the symptoms of ADHD and Dyslexia was huge. Many parents are worried about ADHD and dyslexia. So, again, it just works.

We stumbled upon the autism one by mistake. One of our docs has a passion for wanting to work with autistic children. We did this advert and it worked extremely well – 50 people in the room and they loved it.

It got people into our offices and then we offer them opportunities to continue with us in some way, not to cure autism, but when they understand how chiropractic can help them it changes there perspective on how they can benefit.

It takes a concerted effort to ensure a high show up rate.

We're going to go through in detail how to run the campaigns to drive people to your events in a later chapter.

The most we've had was over 60 people to actually show up to the day. That's very rare. If you could consistently get 10 people, that's perfect.

The reality is with an ad spend of about $150 to $200, you could pretty consistently get 10 people in the room. Most people will be like, "Oh, it's not worth my while," etc., but with a spend of $150, that's nothing compared to your lifetime value.

You are going to close 50 percent of the room at least. It's absolutely worth it. If you just do this maybe once a month, you have a beautiful source of new clients that you can repeat over and over.

Step #2: Getting Them to Show Up

Getting them to show up is very important. Show up rates can vary. We have pretty consistently shown a 50 percent show up rate, which we have been told by expert is very high.

We have actually achieved 80 percent before but in many industries a 20 percent to 30 percent show up rate from online to a physical event is considered normal.

It takes a concerted effort to ensure a high show up rate. Do not assume they will show up if you're not actively making the effort to ensure that they will show up. You really have to work hard to get them there.

You have to do something really special to ensure they show up. Some type of immediate response after registration is useful. For example, one of the tools we us is Eventbrite, which I love because it's very low tech, very low learning curve, easy to get going straight away.

You get a notification straight away, they get a notification straight away that they're registered in the thank you page.

If you can just do something almost immediately, it's massively going to increase the chances of show-up.

Email confirmation reminders, text reminders, phone call reminders. The key to all those reminders is if you do not get a response from them, you need to go "overboard".

The thing is you might worry that you're going to irritate them but the reality of the situation is that without it, most of the time don't show up if you haven't had some type of contact with them.

Most of the time, do more than you think is appropriate and you'll get a better response than most practices will. Most of the times you'll get away with it and all it will do is increase your show-up rates.

The big thing is just being super apologetic and be super empathetic in your messages and voice messages. Don't be like, "I've been trying to get hold of you." You should be like, "I'm so sorry to bother you. I feel so bad about this. I just really want to make sure that I get in contact with you."

There are a couple of strategies we use to massively increase show-up rates.

One of these is what we call an "ethical guilt trip." We say to people who register that we are putting together a special bag of goodies just for them, which is going to be waiting for them when they arrive.

So, after someone registers, we leverage that in every contact we can, whether it's a text, email or phone call. Our experience is that this makes them more likely to show up.

This also does something very important by also leveraging the law of reciprocity, as Robert Cialdini explains in the book "Influence." It means that we human beings, if someone does something nice for us, we feel obligated to do something back for them even if we don't consciously realize it.

The other strategy we use is getting them to do anything before they come in. They can fill out a survey using Survey Monkey or Google Forms. For example, "It's awesome to have you registered. I want to make sure we give you the most value for the day so please tell us what two questions you would you love to have answered on the day"

All those questions are really important. They also help you prepare for the talk.

The fact is, if you can get them to do anything before they come in, they are more likely to show up.

Step #3: Give Value

It's very difficult for me to give you the full rundown of what you should be talking about in your events and what you shouldn't be talking about. But I promise you, you are more than qualified to do this incredibly efficiently.

You really do not have to worry about what to talk about. If I were to give you one piece of advice, it's that less is more. Stick to talking about three things, or just three main points.

**It's not about the content of what you are going to say.
It's all about the context.**

Most of the time people don't remember what you said in the talk anyway. So, when you talk about too many topics… and I've made this mistake many times… they just really don't remember much of what you say. That's just human nature.

So, you've really got the content down. You don't have to worry about that. How to structure the talk and how to stand up in front of people and talk, that's a training all on itself, but I'll leave you with a few tips right now.

Just go there and honestly try give value on the day. I'm going to go back to what I said earlier – the customer is the hero, we're just the guide.

So, don't go and shove every single green book statement you can find down their throat within the first 30 seconds. They registered for something to help them. You're a dealer in hope, as a leader, that's what you're doing.

You're giving hope that there is an alternative and the key word is seed. You want to seed little cool results you've had with an autistic child, with someone with ADHD, etc. You just meet them where they're at.

I'll just leave you with this. I want you to remember that it's really not about the content. I have been on so many public speaking seminars and trainings … including arguably the guy who's influenced more people on stage than anyone on the planet, I personally was coached by him … and you know, when you get in front of these guys, they all tell you the same thing. It's just not about the content of what you are going to say. It's all about the context.

When I say context, this is what I mean. It's when they walk into the room, how the room looks and how the chairs are set up.

Theatre style is best and, if you know you're going to have 20 people show up, don't have 25 chairs. You always want less chairs than registrants. By the way, this is also applicable for you going into a company.

If you know there's definitely going to be 30 people in the room, make sure there are 25 chairs and then you can stack chairs on the side.

If you're talking theatre style, block the last two rows, because when people walk in, they are more likely to sit in the back row. That kills your energy in the room.

This stuff really matters. I know that sounds small, but context matters.

Have music playing when they walk into the room. That's massively important.

If you go to any top conference by guys like Tony Robbins, T Harv Eker, they never walk into a room without music playing in the background. It's important to have upbeat music.

This is an opportunity to bond with you and your team. Don't just leave them sitting there.

When I walk into practices, sometimes my practices included, and I see 20 people waiting for a talk and no-one is talking to them, I just cry inside at the opportunity we are missing.

Remember, to be interesting, you need to be interested. Just have a conversation with them and the major thing is get them to participate in the talk.

When you're doing a talk, the rules of conversation apply. Meaning that if I ask a question to a group of people, I expect a reply. It's just the rules of conversation. You're just having a conversation with more people.

So, it's not about the content, it's about the context.

Step #4: Convert Attendees to Clients

This is the most important part of this entire chapter because you need to know how to convert people so that they come into your office, so they can get better.

The worst possible thing that can happen when you finish your talk is that you rock the talk, it was amazing, the information was incredible. Literally people are high-fiving you. There's a standing ovation etc. They come to you and they pat you on the back and say, "Thank you so much for such a great talk doc. You're amazing." And then they leave.

That is the worst thing that can happen. While it's great for our egos, it simply does nothing for the client, for chiropractic or for our practice. There is no point in doing it. No one takes action and ultimately nobody gets helped.

You can give them valuable content. But we know we are chiropractors. We get hands on people. That's what we do.

So, here's the golden rule: Never stand up in front of any group of people without making an offer.

Whether it's in a webinar, a talk, or a talk in the office, always make an offer.

Never stand up in front of any group of people without making an offer.

By an offer, I mean at least capture leads. For example, if you get to speak at a Rotary and you're uncomfortable making an offer, you can offer one of your reports. They're not as powerful as making a proper offer, but at least go, "Hey, if you find this useful, write your email down and I'll send you this."

If you walk away from this and decide, "I'm never allowed to stand up in front a group of people without making an offer in some way, shape or form," you will look back at all the clients you have got and money you made by following that one statement and, I promise you, that in itself is six-figures.

Never stand in front of group of people without making an offer. You have a moral obligation to give chiropractic to the masses and, to do that, here are the two main close options:

- **Talk and Screening:** This is very powerful. You do a talk and all you do is set up a scenario where they need to find out more. Let's say you talk about posture and the only way to find out if your posture's good is to have this test. So, you're just teeing it up for the screening straight afterwards.

- **Talk and close:** This is called platform selling. It's a real art. I can be very intimidating. I've probably been in the room for over a thousand closes or performed many closes myself and I honestly believe the one I'm going to teach you right now is just by far the one that gives the most consistent results and makes it really easy.

Voucher Close

Our newest graduates, two months out of practice, do this and close 50 percent of the room. They're really nervous, they've never spoken in front of an audience and they close 50 percent of the room with this.

Many of my experienced docs are closing 80 percent of the room with this. So, we got 30 something people to show up, 80 percent of the people went and bought the voucher.

To make this work, you need to have a printed voucher and you want the voucher to have a value as opposed to just saying, "50% off." You want that total value to be as high as possible. Though you would also state "You save $80," so they realize subconsciously that this thing is worth $160.

Now when somebody sits down on a chair before the talk, and they see the voucher, there's a couple of things happening.

One thing is, whether they realize it or not, there are these two processes that have been burnt in their subconscious. One is they see it's worth $160 and it's pretty good and they may even be thinking, "He's trying to catch me out here trying to sell me something for $80."

But part of their mind is going, "Hey, it's not bad for 50 percent off."

They are now tussling with themselves over the $80, especially in comparison to the $160.

What's beautiful about the voucher close is they do this, whether they realize it or not, for a whole 30 minutes. That's why it's important that you get this in front of them before the talk.

There is a very simple voucher close script, which you can use in corporate, you can use in talks and use anywhere. It's very powerful.

You will just outdo any of your neighbourhood chiropractors by using this script and I'll go through the main elements of it here.

- First, when you finish teaching, you are going to thank them: "When you walked in, there were some gifts and goodies in a bag for you. That's just to you to say thank you so much for showing up. It's awesome that you showed up. It shows me that you care about your health. And in the bag is a little gift from us of a voucher so everybody please take out the vouchers."

- It's important that you get everyone to take out the voucher as you just want to explain it to them.

- You explain the offer and it's very important that you mention everything that will happen when they come to your office – they day one consultation, day two the Report of Findings and the other elements.

   Tell them, "You're going to come in and we're going to do full posture assessments and then we'll do some neurological examinations and a full history, and we'll work with you and find out exactly what's going on."

   Maybe throw in your sports therapy or massage in there if you need it.

   Say that's just a gift from you that's worth $160 but because they showed up today, in order to thank them for attending, it's just $80.

- Next step in order to make this transition is to ask a question, "This is just to say thank you, but let me ask you guys a question. How many of you think it's important to get your spines or nervous systems checked at least once in your life?"

   Don't forget you've told them how important the spine is, you've told them how important your posture is for your nervous system.

- Now, stand with your hand up high. They will mirror you, they will do what you do. Then say, "Thank you. I want to do everything in my power to make that possible. So, is it ok if I do something really special for you?" They are all going to say, "Yes."

- Now very important. You will double your close rate by just adding a limiter, for example, "This is only available if you book today", but you have to tell them why there is this limiter. For example, "I really want to be fair to everyone paying full price for it tomorrow." Then you're going to say, "Does that sound fair?" Everyone is going to say that sounds completely fair.

- So, you then say, "Because I want to do everything in my power to make that possible, go to your voucher where it says $80, just cross that out and write $20 instead. If you pay today, you only pay $20."

- Then you've got to tell them what to do and where to register. You have to tell people exactly what to do. "We're going to finish now and then you're going to stand up and go and speak to Mary over there at the back of the room. Mary give us a wave. You're going to register with Mary."

  You have to point that out. This is important stuff. This affects the close rates. "If you want to join us, that's amazing. If not, that's ok. There is no pressure, but if you'd like to join us, we'd love to help you."

Then you're going to finish the talk. I always finish by saying, "Thank you everybody. Please stand up and clap" and then my stupid lame joke is, "That's the only way I ever get a standing ovation," and everyone laughs. It's important to finish your talk on a good note.

Here are some key points to bear in mind.

- The voucher needs to be seen before the talk.

- No questions during the close. If someone asks a question, say, "I'm going to stay and answer questions in a moment."

- They must register in the room. This was one of our big learning curves, and we tested this. You might be tempted to let them leave the room and register at the front desk because it's easier. But you will not close as many people. So, you need the forms in the room and the ability to take the payment in the room. That means you're going to need help. You'll need a CA or somebody at a table at the back of the room.

This subtle stuff makes a difference.

Charity Close

Another close you can use is the "charity close." This is for when you are in a company and they don't want you to charge.

Simply say to the company that you'd like to donate any money taken to charity and ask them their favourite local charity.

STEP #3: HARNESS THE FULL POWER OF EMAIL

––––––––––

In this chapter, I'm going to cover the fundamentals of how we use email in various ways to grow the practice and build relationships with prospects and patients.

We'll talk about how we use it to connect with patients and I'll go through examples of how we reactivated 563 clients from one campaign within a six to eight-week period.

We're also going to be talking specifically about how to write emails effectively and easily.

There is a lot to cover in this chapter so it's split into three parts:

- Email fundamentals

- Email copywriting secrets

- Example reactivation campaign

EMAIL FUNDAMENTALS

Why Email

If I had a penny for every single time in my life that I've heard the saying, "There is nothing more valuable than your email list," I can tell you I'd be a very rich man.

Every single marketing conference I've ever been in in my entire life tells me there is nothing more valuable than your email list.

But the truth is, I just didn't get it. Everyone said, "The bigger the list, the more valuable. You make money every single email you send."

Well, not me. I wasn't making any money when I was sending emails. I didn't know what these guys were talking about.

I heard that so many times for so many years and then it happened. I realized the power.

I'm not joking when I say that I was absolutely panic-stricken when I realized I wasn't doing any of this marketing and we didn't have our own CRM.

I realized how much money we were leaving on the table and how grossly we were neglecting the situation.

When I got it, I was like, "I need a CRM now. I'm not talking to my list."

Honestly, I got a lot of resistance from my team. That included my business partner and my financial director, you name it. Nobody got it.

I don't want to know how much money I lost by neglecting this.

<hr>

They all said things like, "We can already send emails from the operating system we work with. Why do you need a CRM? The CRM costs money. It's a very intimidating learning curve and email is dead anyway." These are all things I was told.

And two years later, I still had no CRM.

I easily estimate, from what we've been able to do with one now, it probably cost me $1 million at least.

If I think about it, it was a good five years that I wasn't using any type of email marketing or speaking to my lists.

As I'll show you in a moment, I've generated 563 reactivations from one campaign, and we're doing a campaign at the moment that's generating 30, 40, 50 reactivations every time we send a group of emails.

I don't want to know how much money I lost by neglecting this.

The reason that I didn't take action for two years, even when I knew the truth, is a sentence that will sabotage all of our growths. Every single one of us has thought it at some point in our careers. And the sentence is this, "My business is different."

"That works for them, but my business is different. I live in Timbuktu. My business is different. It's all good if you live in California, but where I live, it's different."

Another sentence that sabotages our growth is, "I already know this."

When I've been taught something or I'm sitting in an audience, and I find myself thinking, "I already know this," I'm like, "Focus. Knowing is doing." If you're not doing, you don't know anything.

Another one is, "This won't work for me." A lot of times those sentences take us out the game. "That process won't work for me." "They've got a team." "They're bigger than me. That's a sentence that I've struggled with many times.

Another is, "This is obviously for online business. Not me. Not for bricks and mortar."

Those are some sentences that held me back. So, stop for a moment and think about whether any of them are holding you back too.

The Death of Email

People keep on saying that email is dead. Well, here's the thing. I'm going to give you some stats.

- More than 90 percent of adults use email.

- Marketers continue to reap the benefits of email marketing to its worldwide audience, with 59 percent stating that email is their most effective channel for generating income.

- Despite the rise of social messaging apps, still 74 percent of teenagers use email.

- The average deliverability rate of an email is 98 percent. That's not the open rate, or the lead rate, but the deliverability rate is 98 percent.

- Marketers consistently ranked email as the single most effective tactic for awareness, acquisition, conversion, and retention.

- Email is almost 40 times better at acquiring new customers than Facebook and Twitter.

- Research puts return on investment on email marketing better than any other direct marketing channel.

- More than 60 percent of customers would prefer to be contacted by email.

- 88 percent of all marketers say email marketing is bringing them a positive return on investment.

I think I rest my case on that. But I'm going to talk about how it's definitely lost a certain level of its sensitivity, which means you have to deal with email marketing differently, because we get so many emails these days.

CRM Systems

So, you can get started properly with email, you need a Customer Relationship Management system (CRM).

There are so many of them that you could use and this is not the place to go into the advantages and disadvantages of each. Any CRM is better than not having one to just take the plunge and get going.

I'm not going to say you should use a specific one but try to use on of the known ones like Infusionsoft, MailChimp, AWeber, Drip, Constant Contact.

So, if you haven't got one, go ahead and do that. But don't beat yourself up if your reading this and don't have one yet, it took me five years to get one. We had six or seven clinics before I actually got serious about this stuff.

Reasons We Don't Send Email's to Our Lists

I've just told you those statistics. I've told you how important it is to communicate with your tribe, however, the reasons we don't "talk" to our list are extensive but very important to understand.

Because while this book has a lot to do with the "how to," I promise you this… most of the things that I have to get through to get anyone results is the psychology around the fear about marketing.

And the reasons we don't even talk to our lists amongst many things are these.

We don't talk to our list because of the assumption that, if they're not currently active clients, it may mean they're dissatisfied with our service and they don't want to hear from us.

A lot of time we're like, "Well, he hasn't been in for six months. He clearly doesn't like me," and we build this whole fake story up in our head.

Really, most of the time, they've probably forgotten appointments or missed an appointment. They then got so embarrassed that they just dropped off care.

They dropped off the face of the planet altogether. They don't answer the emails. They don't answer your phone calls. And we assume it's because we haven't done a good job.

But honestly that's just not the case. That's one of the reasons we don't talk to our lists.

Reasons we don't "talk" to our list...

1. The assumption that if they are not currently an active client it must mean they were dissatisfied and don't want to hear from me?
2. Feel like you don't have anything of value to say??
3. Time?
4. Fear of judgement.
5. Fear of appearing to be pushy or desperate.
6. Don't want to "irritate" clients.
7. Don't know what to "say" or knowledge in copywriting.

Another reason is we feel like we don't have anything of value to say. What are we going to tell them? What can I possibly put in an email that they want to hear about?

The next thing is time. We don't have the time to do it.

The next thing is fear of judgment. We've got fear of appearing to be pushy or desperate. And we don't want to irritate clients.

Also, we don't know what to say or have no knowledge of copywriting.

Those are basically the key issues that I came up with about why we don't talk to our lists.

But, here's the thing. We had almost 3,600 visits last week and we send more emails than anyone I know.

So, you've got two choices.

- You can email your clients a lot. And guess what? Some people are not going to like it. But you help a lot more people.

- You email a lot less. And guess what? Some people still won't like you. But, instead of being the doc that helped a ton of people that some people don't like, you'll just be the doctor that helped very few people that some people still don't like. You'll just be poorer and help less people.

I promise. It's just part of the process.

Some people are just not going to like you.

Email Open Rates

Next thing I want to talk about is email open rates. Here are some statistics that I looked up.

Business Type	Open Rate
Fitness centres, sports, recreation (e.g. yoga studio, bowling alley, gym)	15.7%
Fitness/nutritional services (e.g. personal trainer, wellness coach)	13.76%
Government agency or services	21.56%
Health and social services (e.g. hospital, elder care, adoption services)	19.66%
Health professional (e.g. physician, dentist, chiropractor)	16.99%

What that means is that more than 80 percent of your emails are not even being read. Think about that for a second. We're so scared to send emails, but over 80 percent of the emails are not being read. This just means that you need to send double.

I know the little voice is going nuts right now. You're all like, "What? Send double?" Yeah. Send double.

From the top marketers on the planet, I get two or three emails a day.

I'm not suggesting that at all. But sending an email a week is nothing in this world, just because we're so desensitized to it. It's just one email a week.

If they don't want to read it, they just delete it. It's nothing. You're not upsetting anyone. Now, I'll tell you this... having worked with many coaches and many of the top achievers on the planet, they'll always say that successful people have the awareness that they need to develop the difficult but necessary skill of becoming thick skinned. Dan Kennedy calls it immunity to criticism. It's not easy.

The truth is, when you send an email, there will be someone that responds and goes, "You are cowboys. Please stop sending me emails."

I promise you that's got nothing to do with you. It's just got to do with where they are in their lives.

Now, this is much easier said than done. But if this is all you get from working with me, it's very important.

You need to have the awareness that if you really want to play a big game, you without a doubt will receive criticism. I'm not going to sugar coat it for you.

You've got a choice. And this is very critical to understand this.

We've either got the choice between the pain of criticism, or the pain of mediocrity.

If that is all you get from me in this book, that will make a big difference. It's just unavoidable. If you want to play a big game, as you climb up the pole, your ass sticks out more, and you're going to get people that are going to throw stones and it's just normal.

We've either got the choice between the pain of criticism, or the pain of mediocrity.

I just want you to know the reason I'm telling you this is that there's nothing you're doing wrong.

We get complaints sometimes. But there's so many people that we help because of this that I refuse to let it get in the way.

So, I just wanted to give you that. You've got two choices. Pain of criticism, or pain of mediocrity. It's whichever one you choose.

Who to Send Emails To

There are basically three groups of people you're going to send emails to:

- Active clients
- Inactive clients
- Prospects.

Prospects are people that have opted in to your opt in campaigns who have not come in yet. Often, it's the same email that's only slightly changed. The reason I wanted to make that clear is to not make it too intimidating for you. It's not three separate campaigns.

Once you get a bit more advanced, it may be three separate campaigns. That's where we are now. But it's basically the same email, and just changing it slightly.

Segmentation

It's important to make clear that not all email lists are made equal. I've had a few people who've listened to some of my advice and they said, " We just went for it. We did a reactivation campaign and I haven't got any results."

I think that, if there's any one thing I can tell you, it's by the end of this, it's impossible for you not to get results. But I also want to emphasise that not all lists are made equal.

What most people do wrong is they just send an email to their entire database. That is not what we do.

Segmentation is so important to this process of being successful. What most people do is they mistakenly classify inactive clients as one demographic. But in reality, not all inactive clients are equal.

These are some of the demographics that you're going to be classifying your lists according to. You've got inactive clients and then you've got to break them down according to the demographics, such as, for the reactivation campaign:

- Age
- Gender
- Number of appointments attended
- How much they spent
- How long since they last came in

You've also got to decide how far back you are going back in your lists.

Sometimes, you might also want to segment out certain sources of introductions. You may not want to reactivate anyone from that weird psychic fair that you went to, for example!

This is the basics of the minimum segmentation that we will do in an audience. If this is all you did, you'll get better results because you are narrowing that group. And you can do more for that group.

We'll go into this in more detail when we look at the example reactivations campaign shortly.

EMAIL COPYWRITING SECRETS

Before we go any further, in my experience, you won't take any action on this topic until you have a basic understanding of copywriting.

As you read this, please know that, in my first year of university, I failed every single first test.

So, I'm certainly no academic, but if I can do so can anyone. But we're going to go through the step by step guide to how to do copywriting and this is all you need to know to get going.

I'm going to give you a warning now. You are going to get bombarded by certain coaches who are going to say, "If you don't know copywriting, you're dead."

Well, here's the thing. We're chiropractors. That means we are adjusting people. I haven't got 40 years in the industry like Dan Kennedy to become an expert at copywriting.

While I acknowledge it's important, remember this is all about becoming good enough. That's all it is. We're going to get you to good enough. And then I'm going to give you a sneaky trick at the end that's going to help you outperform all the "experts".

The Art of Copywriting

We'll start with the art of copywriting – all the basics and a how to guide. This applies to writing copy for any media. Then we'll go on to some specific of writing email copy.

In our marketing office, what we love to do before we have our meetings in the morning is put a little quote of the day up on the board just to get everyone's mind thinking a bit differently.

The quote for you about copywriting is, "Sell a good night's sleep and not the mattress."

Copywriting is the power to put words on paper that produce money.

That just really rings true about how important copywriting is, especially as a chiropractor. You're not so much selling an adjustment or whatever, you're actually selling the service that the adjustment is going to provide and that journey that those adjustments are going to get you to.

Basically, this means that whenever you talk about any form of copywriting, rather than talking about the actual product, it's vital that you're talking about it's going to provide.

One definition of copywriting is that it's a marketer's way of creating an emotional connection with an audience. That can be through emails, blogs, social posts, videos, any content you put out there.

But someone who is a bit more esteemed in the world of copywriting is Dan Kennedy and his definition of it is "The power to put words on paper that produce money."

That's really the most important part of that that you need to remember, especially in chiropractic. The pure power to be able to just write something that produces you money is an incredible power to have. And it gives you the ultimate freedom, power, and security.

Copywriting Steps

Copywriting is basically a step by step process. And we're going to go through that now. This is what you need to do before you attempt to put out any emails or any other marketing material.

The first step is that you need to create a fact sheet. This literally is a piece of paper. You write down every single fact you can think of about your product or service.

That can be the price, how much it is, how long the product's going to last if it's a special offer. What's going to be included with it if it's a package. How many sessions are involved?

Every single thing you think is important about your product, just get it down so that you're not trying to constantly think about what you are providing? Here you've got everything written down. And it's all in front of you.

The second important thing you have to do is create a benefit sheet from that fact sheet. You're thinking about what the benefits of your product are.

You need to remember that a feature and a benefit is a very different thing.

An example is when you think of a car, an airbag is a feature of a car, a wheel is a feature of a car. When you think more deeply into how that feature benefits that product, an example is that the airbag is in there to protect you in case of a car accident.

People don't care so much about what's in something. They care about how that something is actually going to impact their decisions to buy something or be involved with that product.

The next important point is that you need to create your killer offer. This is really important, probably the most important point out of all of these steps.

Your copy can't begin until you know what you're selling. For it to stand out, you really you need to make sure that your offer is the best thing out there and it's different from everyone else.

Copy often works backwards. When we started off our Easter campaign to reactivate some clients back into the clinics, we started by having a meeting to figure out what the product we were going to be putting out there was going to be.

The first question was, "What's the offer going to be? What are we actually trying to get these clients in for?"

Rather than trying to think of how we were going to get them in, we needed to know exactly what we were getting them in for. Because, that was the most important point.

As soon as you have that, you can work your way backwards. Stephen Covey said to start with the end in mind. That's always the way. Backwards is the way forward.

The next step is to create headlines. Try writing down different variations. Because if the headline doesn't grab your attention, then the rest of the copy is meaningless.

Copywriting Steps

1. Create a fact sheet
2. Create a benefit street
3. Write killer offer
4. Create headlines
5. Write a draft first - DON'T EDIT
6. Edit rough spots and style

The headline is that first big thing they're going to look at. When you look at a newspaper, you're going to see that main headline, the big news of the day going on. If that isn't interesting to you, then you're not going to care; you're not going to want to read the article.

As long as your headline is catching and really engaging, then they're going to want to read on.

The next step is to write a draft first. Once you have everything in place, you know exactly what you're going to be writing about and what you're going to be offering.

Don't try and think too much about it. Just get everything you can think of out on to that piece of paper into that email.

Just really just go for it. Get everything out. Pretty much just a brain dump. Because what happens is when you begin to write, your subconscious begins to write for you. And you start getting ideas out and literally it's just a brain dump.

It's also really important to try and write as yourself. Sometimes you'll want to oversell yourself or try and stand out a bit more, so you become something that you're not. But if you're just really honest and you'll just be yourself, then you're going to stand out a lot more than you think you would.

It's really important as well that as you get your first version out that you don't edit it at all. If you start to see red squiggly lines because you made spelling mistakes, leave it. It doesn't matter. Just get everything out there.

Because as soon as you stop, that flow is going to stop. And you're going to think, "Oh, I could probably change that." Then you're going to start going backwards. And not forwards.

The last little important step is once you have that information out, then you can start to make it look nice. You can add in italics. Make things bold that you want to have to stand out. Use underlining too if you want to highlight things that you think are really important. You can use links as well.

When you look at an email, the most important thing is what we call the zig-zag rollercoaster.

When they're working their way down the email, you want them to be going on a journey. They're probably not going to be reading everything there, but we want to make sure that they're making their way down that letter or down that email to get to the most important point, which is that offer at the end.

These things really help them to follow their way through. The things that stand out. They're making their way to each one. They're joining the dots and getting to that point in the end.

Email Copywriting Formula

Let's talk a little bit more about emails specifically now. This is our email copywriting formula. If you follow these steps, then you're going to really make a huge impact with your emails. These are the six commandments of copy.

The first one is a killer subject line.

When you go into your inbox, you have an email, you don't see that email. The first thing you see is that subject line. If your subject line isn't intriguing, or really impacting, then they're not even going to open their email to begin with. That email is pointless.

It's really important that you have a killer subject line. But it's really just as important to remember that it's the more intriguing things that work, things that aren't quite directed to what the email is about but, in some way, can be linked to it.

Email Copywriting Formula

1. Killer subject line
2. Use of personalisation and personality
3. Bullet points
4. Sub-headings
5. P.S's
6. Buttons

Recently we sent out some emails about what's going on with our Inner Circle and there were a few funny subject lines like, "It's National Proposal Day." People think, "What the heck is this?" but they open it because it's intriguing. Then once they get in there, they're thinking, "Oh. Okay. I understand." And then they're in that email.

The next point there is use of personalization and personality. You really want to make sure that you're bringing yourself into that email, you're bringing that personality.

This is especially for reactivation clients because they're going to know who you are. They're going to want to connect with you on a personal level. They're going to want to know that you're you.

By personalization, I mean having their name in there and really making it seem like that email is just for them, rather than sending out a huge batch of emails and having it seem like they're just one of a crowd.

It's really important that actually you're making it seem like that email is just for them.

There's a little statistic as well… automated emails which include personalization have a 75 percent higher open rate than those that don't. If they really feel like that email if for them, then it's going to go a long way.

The next key is bullet points. These really help to break down an email. They help to guide the person reading it through that email too and they help to break down the really important points.

Connecting with that a little bit too is subheadings, breaking off an important point in that email. If you want to kind of begin to segment it into another section of your email, subheadings really help to do that. And they're really a useful thing to use in your emails too.

The next one is the P.S. Statistics have shown that sometimes all people read is the P.S. They will open the email, but they won't look at anything. They'll go straight down, and for some reason they only read the P.S.

You can never have too many P.S.'s. I have seen emails with like seven P.S.'s. It doesn't matter. But sometimes that's all they read. It's just this weird thing that people just do.

When you're using those P.S.'s, it's really important that you use those to your advantage by highlighting the really important points of that email. Because if that's the only thing that they end up reading, then you want to make sure that they get the most vital things.

The things we do is we reiterate the number to call or how long the offer is going on for. We just reiterate those important points.

The last thing there, this is more so to be used especially when you're using a CRM, as soon as we started using buttons in emails, the opt in rate shot up. It's just a really, really cool thing to use.

As soon as you see a big shiny button, you just want to press it. You just want to know what's going to happen when you press it. Even if you don't want what's on the other side of it, the intrigue to press a button is paramount.

Putting a button in there with like, "Click here to get your offer now" really makes a difference. We'll talk about that more in the reactivation example.

If you follow those six commandments, then your email is going to look great.

Seinfeld Emails

Now we're going to talk about Seinfeld. Not the American TV show Seinfeld, it's actually something called Seinfeld emailing. What are Seinfeld emails? Well, to sum it up, the Seinfeld email is pretty much about nothing.

Now you're probably thinking, "How can I send an email about nothing? Why would anyone care about nothing?"

Well, I'm going to tell you the big secret now. You think you have nothing to talk about? Well, actually you do have things to talk about.

You can talk about what happened last week. You could talk about your plans for the holiday season. Or what you bought recently that you regret or what made you angry, but you're laughing about today.

You can talk about a funny thing from the past that taught you a lesson. What you've been eating lately that was tasty or not.

The BIG secret!

So... "nothing" to talk about?

- What happened last week?
- Plans for the holiday season?
- What did you buy recently that you regret?
- Made you angry, but you are laughing about today?
- Funny thing from the past that taught you a lesson?
- What have you eaten lately that was tasty... or not?

Courtesy of Russel Brunson - Author of Dotcom Secrets

All of these things are things that you're probably thinking, "Why on earth is one of my clients that I haven't seen for three months going to care about what happened last week?" But trust me. You may think they're going to find that boring. But people find life interesting.

Something that you may think is nothing may to some people be the most exciting thing they read this week. It's a really, really powerful thing.

This comes from an awesome book called Dotcom Secrets by Russell Brunson. And this is where we found this concept.

I highly recommend the book but the big thing I got from it was this one chapter. I absolutely devoured the book in like two days. But there was one chapter about "Seinfeld" emails. It's based on the idea that Seinfeld was essentially a sitcom about nothing.

When I saw it, I thought, "This is awesome. It takes all the pressure off. I can write emails about nothing."

Let me illustrate how powerful it is with a story. I gave the book to someone in our marketing team and said, "You've got to check this out."

The segment was about two pages. I said, "Read this." Then I grabbed my computer and I quickly wrote an email of an example of a Seinfeld email. It took me not even five minutes. Because I knew he was reading about what a Seinfeld email is, I quickly wrote something down.

When he finished those two pages, I handed him my computer and all I said was, "That's what a Seinfeld email could look like."

Then I walked out of the office and I think I said something like, "We should probably just send that." Then, two hours later, I came back, and I said something along the lines of, "You know what? We should just send that email."

He looked at me and he said, "I've already sent it." And I'm telling you this. I scribbled it just quickly in the amount of time it takes to read one or two pages in a small book. I handed it to him. No editing. No thinking. I never thought he was going to send it.

But, here's the thing, if he had not sent that email, what would I have done? I would have gone back. I would have said, "It's not ready yet." I would have said, "Wait until tomorrow. I'm going to edit it. I'm going to check it again. I want to recheck it. The spelling is not right. And that sounds stupid."

My little voice would be going crazy. Who wants to hear this nonsense that I just scribbled down in five minutes?

Instead, he just sent it. He was really worried when I came back in and he realized that I hadn't intended for him to send that stupid email that took me less than five minutes to write.

But then we looked at the results. In the first 30 minutes of that email going out, we'd already had 30 people opt in to it. The average time it takes normally for people to opt in is maybe a couple of hours, perhaps it takes until the next day for them to have read it when they get in.

But we sent that email and within 30 minutes we had 30 opt-ins from it. We thought that maybe we'd found a good thing here.

So, let me read you some lines. It's so lame!

> *"Hey Jack. It's the New Year. New year's resolutions, new goals, targets and things to be achieved in 2018. If you're anything like me, this is my favourite time of the year. New beginnings just feel really great, don't they? Let me quickly introduce myself.*
>
> *My name is Dr. Ryan Rieder and I am one of the chiropractors at Halsa. I work very closely with Doctor Quinton. (I hope you've been enjoying his brilliant videos.)*
>
> *Anyway, my New Year's Eve began with the mandatory Jools Holland Hootenanny and watching the glorious fireworks over London, on TV of course.*
>
> *I was determined to start the year off with a bang, so on the 1ˢᵗ of January I hit my local gym. But being a bank holiday, all the gyms were closed. But luckily, I got in first thing the next day to smash a great spin session.*
>
> *Wow! How great is spinning? I've managed to keep the spinning going and what a great few days I have had. The last 72 hours have been just as productive as the last three months of 2017.*
>
> *Anyway, I just wanted to send you a quick message to cheer you on at this time of the year. Whatever it is you want to achieve, you can do it.*

We have been inundated with clients at Halsa wanting to start the new year with a bang to get their 'New Year, New You MOT' free treatment. I've been so impressed with everyone taking such initiative and coming in. I think we have already had over 500 people come in specifically for this offer and the expiry date is the 31st of January, so I'm expecting a huge flood in the coming weeks."

You see it's just about nothing. Do you think you can send an email about your gym session? You can do this.

Maybe you just had a funny conversation about your childcare woes. You can write an email about that. The subject line could be something along the lines of, "Isn't finding a nanny a pain in the…?"

The most important thing with it is that someone is going to connect with it out there. Someone is going to have watched the fireworks on TV. Someone is going to have watched Jools Holland. Someone's going to have tried spinning before. Someone is going to have tried to get in the gym and they found it wasn't open.

Every single thing that you're doing, someone out there is going to connect with that more than with an email that's just literally saying, "This is what's going on in the office. Please come in."

Remember, you can do this. Just write an email about absolutely nothing, whatever you do today. Your life is so much more interesting than you give yourself credit for.

What people do wrong is we try and send them the most factual information that we can about chiropractic and people just are not interested in that.

It's just a really powerful way of connecting. Because, rather than just sending an email, you're actually having a conversation with them.

And that's a really important thing to remember. Even though it's not a face to face or a phone conversation, you actually are conversing because they're going to connect with this and they're going to read this and, in their head, they're thinking, "Yeah, I do that," or "Yeah, I think that would be a cool thing to do." It's just really, really cool.

Remember, life is interesting. If you remember that, then you're set.

Copywriting in Action

Let me finish up with a comment that I believe is very important. The reality is you're probably never going to be a copywriting expert. That's just the truth. The goal at this point is just to help you become good enough.

But would you like to know the secret to getting as much as a nine percent response when all the experts are getting four percent?

Well, here it is. This is why I love teaching this. Because every single expert out there is going to tell you that you need to be the best copywriter in the world.

This is huge. I truly believe that this can cover just about any copywriting incompetence or inexperience. It's simply these four steps.

One, simply doing anything. Simply doing anything consistently is going to get you results. Send a weekly Seinfeld email. If that's all you get from this entire book, that you're going to send one email a week, you will have far more people react to that over time.

Number two, always mix up the media. This is where everyone goes wrong. They just think about email campaigns. But that's not how you get results. Always mix the media. You're sending an email, and you're sending a text, and you're doing a phone call to the 50 people that spent over $1,000. Always mix up the media.

Always multi steps. Never one and done. You've got to understand that, in the history of mankind, we've never been exposed to as many messages at one time as we're being exposed to at the moment.

There's even a thing now called double viewership (watching more than one screen at once, such as your iphone while watching TV) that marketers are talking about that is further decreasing attentiveness. That's why you can't send the same amount of emails you used to. You have to send double or triple.

You can't just do email. You've got to do email, text, post and phone because of double viewership.

> I truly believe that these four things can cover up just about any copywriting incompetence or inexperience...
>
> 1. Simply doing anything! (weekly "Seinfeld")
> 2. Always mix up the media (Email, Snail mail, Text, Phone and Facebook)
> 3. Always multiple steps. Never "one and done"
> 4. Always segment the list! (age, spend, number of appointments)

Have you ever watched a movie while you're flicking through Facebook? That means it's changed. We're not just looking at one screen. We're not just being distracted by one screen. We're being distracted by two screens at once. Now you just have to do more.

And always segment your lists. Nobody does this. This is where the power is. Segment your lists… age, spend, number of appointments.

While everyone else is spending years becoming copywriting experts, you can easily match if not surpass their results with these four simple steps.

That's how we got nine percent response in our Christmas and New Year campaign. I'm just going to give you context. We sent 22 emails, five texts and an extra one or two depending on if they watched a video in the email.

There was one physical letter to the higher spends. And we had up to 500 calls to the people that said, "Yes please I would like the offer."

It's good to have a small list. Small lists are powerful. They're responsive.

When I've cut everything down to only send to people who have adjustments, I'm talking about 5,000. When you cut that down, you may be talking 500 or 1,500. This is so manageable for you. We generated over 585 reactivations from a list of 6,300 people. That's a nine percent response rate. All the experts out there say if you can get four percent response rate, that's amazing.

We used to send a Christmas letter every single year, a reactivation letter. Maybe we'd get four percent but often a two percent response from that.

Compare that to this. A nine percent response.

All we did different is we had a CRM, we sent multiple steps and we spoke to an audience. We also thought about, "If they don't respond yet, what are we going to do?"

It's just about planning your campaign out. And it's just unbelievable results.

I tried to post those statistics on a very well-known marketing group for chiropractors, and the guy that runs it, an expert in the marketing field, wouldn't even let me post it. Because he was so scared that the results were so good. And I was only trying to serve the group about using multiple media.

That's how good these results are. I promise you. Just follow the steps. Nobody is getting these results. But it's just because we have multiple steps and media. And we're segmenting. And we're making the time to do the work.

Best Subject Line

It doesn't matter how amazing your copy is in your emails. Unless you have a killer subject line, it won't even get opened.

You could spend hours and hours making your copy absolutely perfect and amazing. But your subject line could be really boring, and it doesn't get opened.

I thought it would be cool to share with you best performing subject lines from the most recent campaigns we've done.

"Got the Christmas Blues, Jack?"

This was included in our Christmas reactivation campaign. We sent that to 4,000 people and 25 percent of the people we sent it to opened that. That was a really good open rate for us.

If you remember, the average open rate for chiropractors, we're within the area of health, was 16, 17 percent. We got 25 percent, that's really good based on that statistic.

"Hootenanny and fireworks done, what's your resolution, Jack?"

This one was also used in our reactivation campaign, coming towards the new year part of it.

That was sent to the same people and it got 1,500 opens. There was more intrigue on that and it got 38 percent of the people we sent it to opened that one.

"Have you seen the news, Jack?"

The last one, which was in the same campaign too, had 4,000 emails sent and 50 percent of the people we sent that to opened that.

That was amazing. Such a basic subject line, but with so much intrigue. Because they're thinking, "Well, hang on. What is the news? I wonder what's going on. Is it something major? Is it something that's going to affect me? I want to know what it is."

The important thing to highlight with all these subject lines is that there's a trend going on. They're all questions.

They're not question in the respect of, "How old are you?" or "What's your name?" They are not something that needs a direct answer.

These are just open-ended questions that really set up a path for intrigue.

People want to know what the answer is. They want to know what's going on. They want to know the news. They want to know what your resolution is, so they can maybe work out what theirs is going to be. It's all about intrigue.

STEP #4: TAKE ADVANTAGE OF PRINT AND OTHER MEDIA

I know that many people see Facebook as the big media that can make a powerful difference in your practice and there is some truth in that.

But before we go there I want to take some time to highlight the importance of other media such as:

- Direct mail and postcards

- Print advertising

- Newsletters

- Text (SMS) messages

Let's look at each.

Direct Mail and Postcards

There are two main ways you can use direct mail or postcards.

- **Cold Traffic:** Sent to people who have never contacted you before, inviting them to a health talk or free appointment.

- **Warm Traffic:** People you have conversed with before, sent as part of a campaign.

I don't really use print media to cold traffic. I only use print, postage, and postcards to warm traffic – people who have conversed with us before. And I'll always use it as part of a campaign. I normally won't rely on it solely.

One of the leading guys in the marketplace at the moment in chiropractic says, "You've got to send a three-step mailer. Don't just send one letter. Send three."

I get it. And I know it's a Dan Kennedy thing. But, why not send a direct mail piece, and email, and a text? The other two are really cheap to do. But the direct mail is so expensive. For me, the mail piece just forms part of the campaign.

I like to send a mail piece to higher value clients. If I've got 5,000 people on the email list, that's already segmented, I'll send them all emails. Then, if people clicked on the offer, I might send them a postcard. For the top spenders, the people that have spent over $500 or $1,000, I'll send those people a letter.

Once you've sent the letter or the postcard, it's just the best thing in the world to follow that up with a phone call. And it's just great justification for the phone call, "Hey. I'm just checking that you got my letter I sent in the post."

Remember, it's just part of the campaign. So, it's just another reinforcement. When you mix media, i.e. print, texts, email, your response rates go through the roof.

We've had people go through an entire email campaign and they didn't respond. So, we sent them a letter in the post and they actually phoned us.

Newspapers

When it comes to newspaper advertising, you need to follow exactly the same copywriting formula we talked about earlier.

We find that advertorial style works the best, where they look like articles in the paper and don't look like adverts.

The newspapers will usually make you want to put a border around it and they'll normally want to put "Advertorial" somewhere. But, anything you can do to get a way to make it look a newspaper piece is what you want.

The mistake that people make with newspaper advertising is they think that people don't read this stuff so they try to make it too short. Usually, it's the more copy the better.

**Of all the sources of introductions, newspaper clients
are the ones that definitely have a higher lifetime value.**

Whether they read it or not, the statistics are very clear. The more writing you have in an advert, the more response you get.

People have tested it to the degree that they put half the advert as a picture, and they literally got half the response rate because half their copy was gone.

I don't know why it works. It just does. I'm a very simple businessman. If someone says to do it, and it works, I just do it. I don't think.

As I've said before, the best type of publications you can advertise in are local – your church newsletter and your local publications.

For me, the highest cost per lead of all my marketing that I've experienced is in newspaper advertising. I have done adverts where it's ranging right up to $200, $300 cost per lead.

I don't do too much of it now but I just wanted to give you a bit of information about it.

Having said that it's a higher cost per lead, if you know the lifetime value, it still might make sense for you.

Because, of all the sources of introductions, newspaper clients are the ones that definitely have a higher lifetime value.

Even though less of them respond, their spend is without a doubt much higher. The conversion rate is going to be higher.

You may spend $400, $500, $600, $700 and three people might respond, but they're very valuable.

Where this really becomes a real option is, if you are the type of doc that is very comfortable selling care plans. Because your velocity of return is almost instant. Your conversion is going to be amazing. If straightaway you're selling a $1,000 care plan, you've got all your money back within two visits.

But if everyone's paying per visit the velocity of return can be very slow and you may end up with a cash flow challenge.

But I just wanted to set context on newspapers, is it something you need to consider? The only thing I can tell you is test, test, test, test.

But I can give you the peace of mind that are statistics. There's very robust statistics that do show that newspaper clients spend more than almost any other source in introduction I have ever seen but your velocity of return is slow. But if you sell plans, absolutely test them.

Newsletters

Next, we're going to talk about newsletters. This is probably going to be the piece that I teach that's going to be the most surprising to you. Because I can honestly say that a newsletter is one of the best overall media that there is.

It's an opportunity for your clients to feel like they belong in a community.

Newsletter Advantages

- Newsletters are perceived as a publication NOT advertising
- Builds trust
- Builds relationship
- Credibility ("EXPERT" in your community)
- Helps build "brand"

Newsletters are not perceived as advertising. This is very important. They build trust. They build relationships. And they also give you credibility because it makes you automatically the expert in the community when you publish a newsletter.

It helps build your brand but the most impressive thing about a newsletter is you get to demonstrate as much as possible without it coming across as advertising.

Let me give you an example. You get to demonstrate patient success or client success, the miracles you had, client of the month. This is all advertising however, as it's put in a newsletter, it's not perceived that way.

You'll also get to show off your referrals. You can have a section in your newsletter that says thank you to referrers, making them feekl special.

Welcome to the new members. You put a welcome to new members in your newsletter. When they open that newsletter, and they see 30 or 40 names on there, it's powerful social proof.

Do you want to eat at an empty restaurant or do you want to eat at a busy restaurant? You want to eat at a busy restaurant. Social proof. People come here.

An impressive thing about a newsletter is that it has one of the longest shelf-lives of almost any media.

Often when you get a newsletter, you put it on your fridge and it lies around on the kitchen table forever. This is what people take home and it lies on the kitchen table for weeks. People also pass it along to others. That's the big thing around newsletters.

So, should you do a print newsletter, or should you do an email newsletter?

An e-newsletter honestly, it's a bit old school now. Almost no one that's successful online does this anymore. It's low cost but at the same time low rewards.

Print Newsletter

- Without doubt more powerful than email
- Still the best way to CONSUME large amounts of information
- Better media to develop relationships
- Always use envelope if you can
- 4 pages feels like a publication
- Use email to supplement print

You can deliver to a lot of people, but do they get opened? You're going to need very strong subject lines for them to get opened.

Nothing builds a relationship like print. A printed newsletter is without doubt more powerful than email.

It's still the best way to consume large amounts of information. It's a better media to develop relationships.

Always use an envelope because it feels like it's got value.

Even better than just using an envelope is if you can write their name and address on it in handwriting.

Four pages at least feels like a publication. And you can use email to supplement it.

Newsletter Content

What goes in a newsletter? First, at the top, a masthead or name for your newsletter. Ours is called the Halsa Gazette. Then a tag line like, "Helping you stay healthy."

The opening article is essentially your Seinfeld article. You can literally take one of the emails that you wrote and just dump it in there. Your opening article is super personal.

A table of contents makes it feel like it's a publication. If you want to make an offer, you can add an insert into the newsletter as opposed to having it in the newsletter. We put it in the newsletter, we make a small offer on each page. But you can just insert in there.

Remember the main purpose is to build our brand. Referrals, social proof, build relationships and you can gain a lot of credibility.

The key to success is consumption. Here's the thing, it's like the emails, if it's not getting read, there's no point. This is where everybody makes the biggest mistake.

The single biggest key to consumption is no more than 40 percent relevant information.

This is the biggest thing that I try to untrain from chiropractors. People are just not as interested as you may think they are about ITB syndrome. They're just not.

The rest of the content is made up of semi-relevant and non-relevant. Therefore, over half of your newsletter is non-relevant and semi-relevant.

Semi-relevant information is made up of the following: welcome to new clients; customer spotlights; employee spotlights; team spotlights; team member of the month; questions and answers.

What goes in a newsletter

- Name or masthead (The Halsa Gazette)
- Tagline
- Opening article (Personal and Conversational)
- Table of contents
- Make an offer – sometimes better as an insert rather than in the newsletter
- Purpose – build brand, referrals, social proof, relationship and credibility

A good tip for this if you've ever attended a webinar before where they sell to you at the end, they take questions and answers at the end, but the questions and answers are often not real. The questions and answers are very specifically put there to deal with objections that they know that the buyers are going to have.

The reason I tell you that is you may have, in your questions and answers, things that you know are concerning your clients. Like, "Can adjustment hurt me? What are the pops and sounds?" That's questions and answers. It's an opportunity to educate.

Next is testimonials. Remember what you say means one thing. What someone else says about your product means everything. It's at least a thousand times more powerful what someone else says about your product than what you say about it.

You can also use this to highlight any other services if you have them. For example, if you do massage, they may not know that. So, highlight any other services or products you sell in the newsletter.

Non-relevant information that goes in a newsletter is jokes, crossword puzzles, quotes, calendar items, photos, photos of celebrities, big charity stuff, contests, and seasonal themes. I'm going to say be very careful with seasonal themes.

Semi-relevant and non-relevant is at least 60 percent of your newsletter. No more than 40 percent relevant content.

Value of a Newsletter

Is it worth doing a newsletter? The answer is yes. But it has to be consistent to get results. Monthly.

Posting it is expensive. The options are to hand it out to your active clients. Fulfilment houses will do this. Printing houses will do this. They'll already stuff it.

You can just hand it to people when they come in. You save a big cost and we have done this before.

Now, remember the importance of segmenting. You might just want to send to all your clients. But, once you do the segmenting, you may see there's only 100 or 200 clients that spent over $1,000 and decide to send them a newsletter every month because you want to keep those.

Remember the 80/20 rule is that 80 percent of your turnover is going to come from 20 percent of your clients. You might think that that is just a rule for other businesses but when we did the statistics, 70 percent of our turnover of $10 million came from 30 percent of our clients.

Crazy. Think about that for a second. $7 million came from just 30 percent of our clients. That's happening in your business too. So, identify those top spenders and look after them.

Tricks of the Trade

Here's some tricks of the trade to make this achievable because I know you're probably not going to do this. Why? Because I'm living proof. We struggle as a team to produce a monthly newsletter. I know some of you have lost interest already and going, "I just can't produce all this content."

But here's what I want to tell you. Here's the cheat sheet. Make the newsletter evergreen. We've done this. Make a few. Just make one. But make sure it's generic.

That means don't put a date on it, don't say this is the August edition. Put Volume 13, Volume 29, volume whatever, instead of a date. That means you can use it over and over.

Be careful about making the opening article seasonal. That might seem easier but don't make it seasonal. If it's a Valentine's Day theme in the opening article, you can't use it in Christmas.

So, don't make the opening article seasonal unless you're going to do it every month.

If you do that, I promise you you're going to show positive return on investment, but I work with chiropractors all the time and I know you're probably not going to do this.

If you make one, at least you're doing something. Even if all you did was posted your newsletter to every single new client, with all the demonstrations in it, referrals, new clients, a picture of you with celebrities before they have their Report of Findings. Do you think that your conversions are going to improve if you have the opportunity to show them proof of your product? Without a doubt. So, this is something that I highly recommend doing.

I can't not teach you this. Because there's going to come a time in all your careers when you're going to go, "Okay, what's the next step for us?"

I've done this many times and it's not about the new thing. You forget things that you learned. And you go, "You know what? I need to produce a newsletter monthly" and you'll be ready for it. But you might not be ready yet.

When you've got your newsletter, you can put it at the front desk, you can send it out to new clients. It's important stuff.

Text (SMS) Marketing

I quickly want to talk about text marketing also. This is very powerful. It has the highest deliverability of any type of media and highest open rate of any type of media.

But be careful with it because people do regard texting them as quite a personal space. We've learned this lesson. We sent one text and it literally caused Bedlam in my office.

The text was for clients who never came for day one. I tried to reactivate them. I sent like 100 of them a text that said, "I've been trying to get in touch with you about your upcoming appointment."

They go, "What upcoming appointment? What's going on?" The phones are going off the hook. Everyone was like, "What have you done?"

But that's how you test. Next run we went a little softer. But look how powerful that is.

Then it's best when used as a follow up to an email. I like to send a text when someone clicks on something or to all the higher spend groups. Just be very apologetic in your text and emails. Lots of empathy. And most of the time it's open-ended stuff like, "Did you get our email? Did you get our letter?" or "We tried to call."

Broadcast texts do get read. However, open-ended texts are much better. It's just there to start a conversation.

There are some fancy pieces of tech that will link directly into your CRM and are also two way, meaning if they respond it shows up on your computer or ipad etc.

Text marketing

- Highest deliverability rate
- Highest open rate
- Be a little careful with frequency as people perceive getting a text as quite a personal thing
- Best when used as a follow up to an email or letter (Did you get our email? Did you get our letter? We tried to call.)
- Broadcasts do get read but most powerful is open ended texts and questions
- Start a conversation (best is two way options)

We can send 100 texts and I can respond to them live like Facebook Messenger or chat. But it's on a computer. It's awesome. We're actually having conversations with people.

But, I'm going to tell you your biggest bang for your buck in your clinic right now... I know that you can send texts from a lot of your systems, but I would recommend this. Just have a cheap mobile at the front desk and get your team to start sending more texts.

I know a very successful clinic, they purposely choose to send a text via a telephone, by a mobile, instead of using a big fancy system.

I know what you're thinking, "It's extra work." But, really is it? How many new clients can you possibly have in a day? If you've got 10, it's a lot.

But, on average one, two, three a day and it's like, "Hey, it's Mary at the front desk. I'm checking, are you coming in for your appointment? I just want to confirm. " Make it as personal as possible.

Your show up rates are going to go through the roof and you're going to connect more with your clients. It's the biggest bang for your buck. Just suck it up. Put a mobile phone at the front desk. And get your team to text a bit more. And you will have awesome results.

Remember this the new lead is a conversation. This is what everyone is talking about. You've got to converse with your audience.

Text messaging is a great start of a conversation. And it can be done easily and effectively simply by a mobile phone at the front desk without worrying about complicated software.

STEP #5: MAKE THE BEST OF FACEBOOK

In this chapter, we're going to cover Facebook. It is very powerful and exciting, and it can give you huge rewards very quickly.

But my warning is that Facebook is a fast-moving, fleet-footed elusive beast.

The rules literally change daily. That's not just a figure of speech. Literally, Facebook changes certain rules daily, which makes it very difficult to keep up with what you can do and what you can't do. Equally it makes it difficult for me to "teach" you how to tactics in the format as it changes so rapidly. I will however to my best to give you a overview.

So, there's a few options to enable you to be successful with Facebook.

- Be in it like we are, doing ads every day, testing and trying things so you learn from doing it.

- Pay to be close to someone who is "in it": You can work with someone that's doing it every day and learn from their experience.

- Pay someone to do it: You just pay a specialist to do it for you. (I am not a fan although there are exceptions to the rule)

I've explored all these options at different stages and there are pros and cons to each depending on where you are in your business. But essentially, you have to find a way of either being the expert on being alongside someone who is.

The Myth of Simple Solutions

It's no coincidence that I am teaching Facebook strategies towards the end of the book. The reason for that is I wanted to introduce you to Ryan's inconvenient marketing and business truth.

You're not going to like what I'm going to say now but it's one of those truths that was told to me very early in my career.

The problem is that chiropractic owners, and business people in general, waste much time and energy and emotion desperately searching for a single, simple solution, or quick fix, to complex problems and opportunities where a simple solution may not exist.

Honestly, I would actually love to pay someone just to do every single bit of marketing for me. I have had quotes as much as $10,000 a month to do that.

I've tried them by the way, and it was horrific. I have done everything you can possibly think of, and I think my biggest lesson... and the reason I was so determined to talk about screenings and talks and all that first... was the simple, single solution doesn't exist.

For some, Facebook is the single, simple solution. It's scary to think how many businesses are so reliant on Facebook, and it's even scarier to think that one day Facebook may not exist.

That's why I'm so determined to have a robust business so that I am ready for that day when Facebook doesn't exist or there's a new Facebook. People have already started leaving Facebook a little bit. Kids don't use Facebook as much anymore.

It's just important to recognize that one day Facebook may not exist, but we'll still have emails, we'll still have phone calls, we'll still have shopping malls, we'll still have gyms and post. We'll still have all those things. We'll still have internal referrals, we'll still have newsletters.

Often, we're so focused on looking for the simple, single solution that we miss the diamonds right under our nose.

But, when someone else controls the media, it's a little bit scary because at the end of the day, you may have a big audience on Facebook, but it can be taken away overnight.

I've seen it happen. We've got a massive viewership on Facebook now that we can re-target, but that can be taken away from me tomorrow.

If we do something that pisses Facebook off, they can shut down our account, and many people have had their accounts shut down for trivial things. It's just important to remember that. There isn't a single, simple solution.

Often, we're so focused on looking for the simple, single solution that we miss the diamonds right under our nose.

Most of our bankers and diamonds we have covered in previous chapters already. I did not build my business on Facebook. I built my business on the streets, in gyms, in malls, in supermarkets, doing internal referrals, doing competitions, sending out newsletters, sending out emails, getting on the phone.

Our $7 million business was built like that. It was not built through Facebook.

But, having said that, Facebook has certainly helped us add another element to our business and it's very important right now.

So, we're now going to talk about Facebook, why it's important and what you need to do to make the most of it – including some specific strategies that are working well right now for chiropractors.

I think at this point in the New Patient Avalanche System, you've got a good enough understanding of what we're trying to do here. You know that the fortune is in the follow up and it's about multiple forms of new clients.

Now, by the end of this chapter, you should have the basics to be able to run your own Facebook campaigns.

Many people start out on Facebook with a feeling of anxiety, frustration and fear. I hope that if you're one of these people, this will make sense.

Hopefully, you'll finish this chapter a lot more confident about how to use the Facebook platform without the fear.

Why Facebook Matters

Let's start with understanding why you should care about Facebook.

The big attraction is its potential reach. At the time of printing of this book, facebook has a worldwide audience of more than 2.3 billion monthly active users – a 14% increase year over year. That's 30% of the planet's population! There is a good chance your target audience is within that.

It is also an important part of the life of users. Users access Facebook eight times a day for up to 20 minutes at a time. There are 1.74 billion mobile active users, an increase of 21% year over year.

One of the first things users do every morning – before nourishing and hydrating themselves or acknowledging their partner – is check Facebook. For large numbers of people, they switch off the alarm, and just start scrolling.

Marketing Benefits of Facebook

- The power of **targeting** is worthy of a super hero!
- **Access communities** more efficiently than other social media platforms.
- Unheard of **speed** at which you can access that community.

Every 60 seconds on Facebook, 510,000 comments are posted, 292,000 statuses are updated, 136,000 photos are uploaded, and 300 new profiles are created.

It's clear you have a growing and very engaged audience.

So that's the big picture about Facebook but let's go into some of the reasons why it can be so important for your marketing.

One of the big things about Facebook is that it has power of targeting worthy of a superhero.

You're targeting not everyone, but someone. You can get your message only in front of the exact ideal audience you want within a specific distance from your establishment.

That's the most powerful thing about Facebook. It is crazy easy to target.

The next key factor is the ability to reach communities more efficiently than with other social media platforms.

With some Facebook groups, you get to spread awareness of your product to people who need your product, but do not know it yet.

The speed at which you can access that community is unheard of. Within 15 minutes with Facebook, you can get a message to the mothers of your town, who are interested in their health, live within 10 miles of your clinic, and are above 30 years old.

When we look at Facebook, an analogy I like is that it's no different than a screening. Because you have to be present at a location where people are browsing with no specific agenda. You have to stand out from the mass, get noticed and get to engage with them.

Then you educate them to serve the person and also have a bit of reciprocity, so they make an intelligent decision to do business with you

You talk to them, you educate them so they're not what we call a 'cold lead,' and it's an intelligent and easy decision for them to do business with you.

If they like your product and they think it's right for them, you then give them the opportunity to make the first step to becoming a client of yours.

At a screening, it's basically exchanging information, purchasing a voucher and getting on the phone with them.

On Facebook, it's no different – exchanging details, email, phone numbers, "I'll get in touch with you and get you booked." The set-up is identical.

How to Use Facebook

The power of Facebook is that it can be adapted to a plethora of ad objectives. Here are some of the ways you can use it.

Number one, workshops. A workshop is a simple ad that redirects to a opt in page (click funnels, leadpages, Eventbrite page). Eventbrite is an easy way to get going because it is free, where your audience gets to submit their details to opt in.

The reason why it's a great place to start is because you're using a third party, which means that the lead will have to go through an extra hoop, which means the lead will be hotter. The person has put a lot more effort into giving them your details.

How to use Facebook

- Workshops
- Lead/New Patient Generation
- Passive Re-targeting
- Active Re-targeting

If your not charging to attend the talk (we don't) then Eventbrite doesn't charge you for that. It allows you to get friendly with the platform and get potential good results from a campaign like that.

Next, new patient lead generation – people that directly exchange their personal details through Facebook in exchange for information or an appointment at your clinic.

The cool thing with that is you can get quick results and traction through an ad campaign like this.

The only problem is that it's all stuck within the Facebook environment, meaning that you don't get an automatic notification/email when someone opts in without a third party plug in. So while it absolutely can get you going very fast and you will get traction, the process is quite cumbersome to manually log in and check your leads to contact, and again without a third party plug in there is no automatic follow up or email that happens directly after someone fills in the form. This also becomes important when your looking to call them or contact them as soon as possible after they have filled in the form on Facebook. Statistics show that the speed at which you follow up or call them, massively increases uptake of the said thing

The unforeseen disadvantage is that they don't go to a separate page meaning that while you may get a lot of opt ins, the quality of the lead may not be as high as if they had had to go to the extra effort of having to go to a separate page and fill in their details. Its almost too easy at times which can sometimes be a bad thing. They just have to press a button, their details fill up immediately, and press another button and they're done.

It's very easy for them to forget about your product, but you generate leads really quickly and we've had great results from these campaigns.

Next, passive retargeting – this is a powerful way for you to push more content to more engage the audience. For instance, if a member of your audience watches one of your videos on Facebook, you can re-target them based on what they watched.

If someone has watched some of your video, there is engagement there. They're intrigued. You can target those people. Everything they do within an ad is captured by Facebook and you can re-target them specifically.

People who watch the video all the way through, those people have enjoyed the content, they're very curious. Those are the kind of people you want to push a lead generation ad straight away because they're hooked.

Finally, active re-targeting. This is an advanced strategy to close audiences who have taken decisive steps in your funnel but did not complete the objective.

What that means is that if for instance, you have a workshop or a health talk that's coming up, someone clicks on the link, drops on the Eventbrite, and just doesn't apply.

They're engaged. They've seen your ad. They've seen the image. They've stopped by. They've read your copy. They're interested. They went on the landing page, read the information there, and just didn't follow through.

Those people can be re-targeted even though they left the Facebook environment, they went onto a third party, you can still re-target them.

Tips for Facebook Success

Now, let's look at some tips for how to succeed on Facebook, taking into account that, as I said, Facebook has rules that change daily.

At the moment, this is what Facebook is looking for in order for its algorithm to push your ad higher to more people. If you play by those rules, your ad will perform great.

First, Facebook will prioritize the user to the advertisers. It's common sense. Without the users, Facebook is nothing.

They will push for you to have a friendly user interface. Facebook is starting to penalize click bait – people who just cut out a piece of the title just for you to click on it and that's not being helpful for the users. It's being quite inconvenient. There are a few strategies you can implement to help with that.

What Facebook Wants

- Facebook will prioritise the user to the advertisers
- Facebook wants you to spark conversation and engagement rather than pure "Click" and "Lead Gen" Ads
- Human to human conversation: Don't try to make it look professional, slick and polished. Be human and personal.

Facebook wants you to spark conversation and engagement rather than the pure click or lead gen ads.

I've already talked about "Conversation is the new lead." So, what's conversation? What's engagement on Facebook?

It is exactly what you think. It's people commenting in the comment section. It's people sharing, liking, tagging each other.

When Facebook sees a post that creates a lot of engagement and conversation happening on a specific post, it will push it higher because it sees the users are enjoying this specific content.

It has to be human-to-human conversation. Don't try to make it look professional, slick, and polished. Be human and personal. People buy from someone, not the company.

That's a really important point. We are seeing that the more "amateur" the video, the better your results, the better the engagement.

Because people are scrolling on Facebook just looking for pictures of friends, family, cats, and if you have a stock photo, you know it stands out. But it stands out in a negative way. They know it's an ad.

If you blend in with that, but stand out at the same time, that's what Facebook is about. What works is amateur pictures that stand out.

It's worth knowing that Facebook pages with smaller followings generally have higher reach and engagement rates. That's very good news for an industry like chiropractors.

For pages under 1000 likes, the reach was 22.8% and the engagement was 14.21%. If you go up to 500,000 and a million likes, you get 7.4% and 11.7%.

The only reason for that is because of engagement and conversation. These big companies who top 500,000 to a million likes don't have the capacity to be able to engage with their audience on a granular level.

The pages that get to engage and generate those conversations are your pages. A comment gets posted, you can have that immediate response. You can communicate with them without using robots or things like that. It's just pure human interaction. That's why this is exciting for us.

Facebook will give you more, add more reach, when it notices a lot of interaction with the posts, comments, share, likes, etc.

Curiosity is the Holy Grail when it comes to a Facebook ad. People start and stop scrolling for curiosity. They ask questions because of curiosity. They click on the link to learn more because of curiosity.

Curiosity is what you need to strive for when it comes to your ad campaigns. Ask questions. Ask to engage. The way you write your copy etc., it all comes down to curiosity.

When it comes down to it, Facebook is a lot more than a social media platform. For us Facebook marketers, it's a huge data base. It captures data like age, gender, income, but more precisely activity on Facebook, such as location and time of activity and scroll time.

For instance, if you like a picture in New York or in Paris, Facebook captures that data and uses that, adds that to your profile. You can then re-target people in your local area based on the location and activity that they're doing.

For instance, if someone is scrolling on Facebook and they pause for a second and then see an ad and scroll past, Facebook will have caught that, and that type of data would be able to optimize your ads.

This all happens in the background. You don't have to worry about, "I want to target people who did this." Facebook's algorithm automatically fetches these people and captures that data and shows them your ad if they think it's appropriate.

It also records events attended and spending habits. If you've ever spent money on Facebook, Facebook captures where you spend your money and at what time of the day you spend your money. So, it pushes ads accordingly to your audience, depending on what your ad goal is.

What's interesting is Facebook also gets third party information. Even if you've never spent money on Facebook before, Facebook goes and buys your spending habits from credit card companies, etc.

Keeping that in mind, bringing this back to the analogy of screening, this makes screening on steroids.

Imagine showing up to your screening venue, and the event organizer stops you at the entrance and says, "Hold on a second. Before I let you in there, who do you want me to let walk around? Do you want men? Women? Both? What age gap do you want? Do you want them to be interested in health, or do you want them to be interested in video games? Do you want them to be interested in reiki, yoga? Tell me what you want."

It's screening on steroids. You can get your message and your ad and your content out there to the people that matter to your business.

You know that if you have that person in front of you in a Report of Findings, you know you're going to close them. Just put that up to them and see how it goes.

But do bear this in mind: Business is a long game and it's a marathon not a sprint.

You're going to be taught some sexy, one-touch campaigns that are going to give you amazing results, I promise you. A lot of them give you crazy, cool results.

But, you will get ad fatigue very quickly, meaning that because we're a local business, if you draw a circle around the people that we can target on Facebook, let's say it's five miles around your clinic, you may only be looking at 20,000 to 30,000 people or less depending on where you practice.

Then you add one or two targets in there and suddenly it cuts down to 15,000 people. Meaning if you try isolate just females or just runners etc it may be cutting down the audience size too much to make an impact.

Now, there's only so many times you can send or show a message in front of 15,000 people to say, "Come in quickly to get your appointment. Special deal!" So, you'll reach ad fatigue very quickly.

The big online markets that advertise on Facebook aggressively often suggest an audience size of between 500,000 and 1000,000 to really get traction on Facebook. So, in our industry, we're talking about tiny audience sizes. There is a limit to the amount of time you can make an "irresistible offer" to 10,000 people around your clinic. People quickly become desensitized to your advert and your cost per lead will climb very quickly.

We've had adverts that when we did them, honestly, we were thinking, "Jackpot baby, we've made it." Then, that same advert, within weeks, all of a sudden, your cost per lead climbs up to $100. I've learned this lesson the hard way.

Our cost per lead at the start was like $5, $15, $20, which is acceptable. Then, all of a sudden, it climbs up to $100 cost per lead, like overnight, because you reach ad fatigue.

By the end of this chapter, you'll know the sexy Facebook strategy, but I'm going to tell you, just be careful. You can't just rely on this strategy or else you will be in trouble with Facebook long term.

Remember, this is a long-term game. You can't be a one trick pony on Facebook or you'll have a tough time.

Now let's look at how to use Facebook in practice.

Kicking Off Your Facebook Campaign

In this segment, we're going to look at the key steps involved in setting up your very first Facebook Ad Campaign.

The correct strategies change ever frequently on Facebook, so it's important to mention that this guide to set-up your campaigns may well have changed at the time of reading this BUT I decided to include it anyway as I believe it may still be beneficial. I have also included a link below that will house a consistently updated basic run-through of the platform. I highly recommend following the link and watching the guided "tour" and tutorial of the platform to get you going, **just visit npamarketingbook.com.**

Let me also just mention that the example below is just one option of a plethora of strategies available to you on the Facebook platform. I do like teaching this basic structure first because it often gets really great results straight out the gates and gets you familiar with playing around on the platform BUT be warned that you cannot win at Facebook long term with just this strategy. The below example is basically a *one touch "offer" advert* which will reach advert fatigue very quickly if you are not mixing it up but it's extremely helpful to get you going.

We like to think it's as simple as 1-2-3.

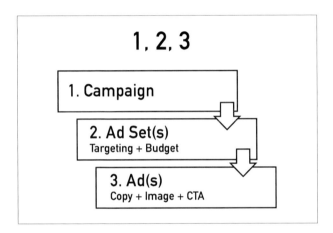

To start with, there's a vital 1, 2, 3 in the little "hamburger" menu to the top left, where it is split Ads Manager, Audiences and Billing.

Then, when you go into Ads Manager, there are 1, 2, 3 main tabs you need to worry about – Campaigns, Ad Sets, and Ads.

1. You start by setting up a campaign. Facebook organises it's ads like you would organise a folder on your computer. You have the big folder at the top, which is a campaign. You could name it "Christmas Health Talks".

2. Within the campaign, you have different "Ad Sets." You can have different ad sets with different targeting, different budgets. Within the "Christmas Health Talks" (for example) campaign, you can have ad sets targeting mothers between 25 and 45, you can target the fathers, and you can just break down targeting.

3. Within those ad sets, that's where you have your actual ad, where you have your copy, the image, the call to action etc.

When you're on the campaigns tab, you can see all your campaigns listed by name and you can dig into them for the campaign details and to check their performance.

If you want to enter a campaign, click on the campaign that you want to look at and then suddenly, you have three little things underneath. 1-2-3.

1. First, you can view graphs and charts, if you're into that kind of thing, just to see how the ad's been performing.

2. Secondly, if there's been a drop or a rise in different metrics, you can edit that campaign.

3. Thirdly, you can duplicate it and rename it, say, "Easter". Just change the copy, change the image, and you're good to go.

Within your campaign, you need to decide your targeting e.g. you might want to target women between 35 and 55 or just men, etc. you also need to set the budgets.

The next element is the ad itself and so you need to create the ad, starting by clicking on the "Create" button.

So, you start with your campaign, establish the ad sets, and then finish with creating your ad.

The elements in creating your ad are as follows:

▪ **Create Objective**: You have to start by choosing an objective. The objective will tell Facebook what you want that ad to do. You have three categories: awareness, consideration, and conversion and each is split into various sub-categories.

These objectives, obviously, will optimize your ad differently.

For awareness, Facebook will just push that message to as many people as you want. This might be relevant for some ad campaigns that you do.

The ad will be pushed to people who are likely, for instance, to click on the actual campaign and go to the landing page. How does Facebook know they are likely to do that? It just knows.

Within consideration, you also have engagement, so for video views, it is pushed to people who are likely to view videos.

For instance, for video views, as soon as you make your ad live, Facebook will have a learning phase, where between 24-48 hours, it's going to push the video to a few people it thinks might be interested.

Then, as people engage, they will look at their profile, "Oh, that person is engaged. What's their profile? I'll push that video to people like that person." It's sort of like a chain reaction.

Also, within consideration is lead generation, which we'll be looking at in more detail here. This goes to people who are likely to give their details to you, while staying in the Facebook eco-system.

- **Audience:** We need to define who you want to see your ads. This may be a brand-new audience or a custom audience. That's where you can use email addresses, phone numbers, etc. to create your own audience.

In defining the audience, we need to define a specific location. By default, it usually specifies your country, which is way too broad.

As you define your audience, you can see your potential audience size. For example, the default is set at United Kingdom, giving an audience size of around 42 million people which is way too high.

If you leave it like that, you'd likely be wasting your money, because Facebook would be pushing that ad to people all over the UK.

So, you can delete that and replace it with something more specific to your exact location. That can cover people who live in this location, people who have recently been in this location, and people traveling in this location.

As soon as you delete the default location, a little world map that pops up, and it gives you the instructions.

Let's say, for example, we are looking at running a campaign for our Windsor office. If I just type in Windsor, Berkshire, United Kingdom, it's still huge. It's an area 25 miles across. The audience is 5,800,000 people. Way too big.

You have distance options, so you can say cities within a certain radius. There is a limit to how small you can make the area, but what you can then do is select "current city only" and drop a pin on top of the city.

You can then repeat that with other locations and drop a pin on them. The beautiful thing about the pin is that you can go all the way down to one mile.

You know that the entirety of your local town or city will be targeted. If there are some other places you want to add, it's the same process.

We can then get more specific about the audience. The default is aged between 18 and 65+, and they're both men and women. In these campaigns, we usually aim for anyone aged 25+. Obviously target audiences can vary but 25 to 65+ is about where we know our clients are going to be engaged with us.

As you specify the audience, you can keep track of how the size changes. If the audience is too large, you need to specify it a bit more.

In order to get the biggest "bang for your buck", you need to go into detail for targeting. This is where the interests and things like that come in. Who's that person that you want to target? Who are those people you want your ad to be pushed to? Who do you want to see your ad?

All you have to do is start typing demographics, interests and behaviours. Once you add something specific, you can see what effect adding that is going to have on the size of your audience.

- **Placement**. Next element is showing your ads to the right people in the right place. So where do you want your ad to be shown?

  For example, you can choose devices, you can choose to only show it to mobiles or desktops.

  You can choose whether or not to show it to people on Instagram. However, it's worth remembering that different pictures will work on different platforms and different copy will work on different platforms. Usually it's best to keep them separate to get a better bang for your buck.

  You can choose whether you want it to appear on Facebook feeds. Often, we want the ads to appear to people scrolling on their Facebook feed but we don't want them on articles.

- **Budget**: The final step in ad sets is your budget. What budget do you want to spend? We usually keep it at a daily budget, depending on the ad. So that's how much money you let Facebook use on a daily basis.

  If you want to run the ad on a specific timeframe, and you want to set a lifetime budget, you can set that up and a little dial comes up for you to schedule when you want the ad to start and finish.

  In lead generation, an ad is useful until it's not, so we usually keep it to a daily budget.

  As soon as you see that you're not getting traction, and you're spending more money than you're getting, that's when you can manually deactivate it.

  When you key in your daily budget, you see the estimated daily reach that will get you.

  So, we went through the campaign, the objective – we set lead generation – and then we went through the ad sets where we selected our audience and the budget.

Creating the Ad

Finally, we come to creating the actual ad. We start by giving it a name and then we choose the format. You can have a carousel ad, a single image ad, a single video or a slideshow. Then you write your copy.

I'm going to work through an example ad – a carousel ad, which has multiple pictures. It's going to be targeted to mothers within the area between 25 and 65+. So, these are mothers who are serious in making changes to their health.

We start by writing in the copy and that's what is going to come up at the top. For us, it's "Limited Availability." That catches your attention, acts as the hook.

We normally use a lot of emojis within the text and what we do is usually Google "emojis" and copy and paste it into there.

Here's the text we add:

"At your local Hälsa Care Clinic we specialise in providing care for those with symptoms that link back to poor posture such as back pain, shoulder pain, knee pain and more. We're giving away 20 discount vouchers to promote our chiropractic offices for a Complete Chiropractic Health Assessment for only £30 (instead of £200). This is a perfect way for anyone to receive care for any of the above or want to improve their overall health... People need to be pain free and adjusted regularly in order to perform their everyday activities to the best of their abilities... We're only giving out 20 discount vouchers this month, so we'll be giving these out on a first response basis!"

If they decide to opt-in they will be informed that Holly will be in contact with them within the next two days. So now we are adding a little bit of person to person, human to human communication. We're making it look very personal.

We're really just saying that there's actually a human that will be contacting them to complete that whole process. The reason we put that on is because the leads are going to be very cold because they're going to stay within the eco-system of Facebook and all they have to do is press on that little button there and they would've opted in.

So, this is just to warm them up, to let them know that there's a human, there's expectations, and it's for a select few, just to build that context around the ad.

Then we add the pictures or cards to the carousel. Depending on which one most click on, Facebook is going to show that card first. You need to choose suitable images and, in our example, we're going to put an image on each card of the doc adjusting.

As well as the pictures, we add text for each.

So, we've got our carousel and next step is to add the CTA (call to action).

You have different options for this, such as "Download, Get a Quote, Learn More, Sign Up, Subscribe."

First, we want them to apply for an actual appointment so we say, "Book Now."

You can see here how the ad looks for now.

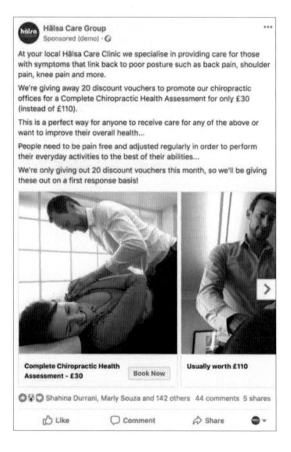

We've got beautiful copy, we've got some beautiful images, we have some call to actions and we have a few headlines.

In addition to the ad, we need to set up a lead form where they would actually exchange their details. This is the last step in the ad creation.

When we start to create the new lead form, we need to give it a name.

There are different types of forms...do you want more volume? Do you want more people to opt in, or do you want them to review steps to give the people the chance to confirm the information?

We want more volume on this type of ad, just so we get an abundance of leads and we can start the following up process. We don't want to add a barrier on this type of ad because when we want to generate leads, we go all out.

We add a headline and usually we add the image from the ad, just so it follows through visually and there's no disconnect.

Next, we add some paragraphs on what the offer is about. This is where all that information lives.

We then have to define the questions or information we want the people to give, such as email and full name. If we want to give them a call, then we need to request the phone number.

You can also add a custom question here such as, "Where's your pain?" etc. We usually keep it blank because we want to keep it simple and we want them to submit their details.

Then you need to define what you want them to see as soon as they press "Submit." That's the "Thank You" screen.

We're going to remind them that, even though they haven't talked to a human, that there's a human here that's going to be in touch. So, we just put more information:

"Holly has received your information and will be in touch within two working days. If you are keen, you can call her by tapping the button below. She's available Monday through Friday from 9:00 AM until 5:00 PM."

That's giving them another option. If they're hot, if they're really wanting to get into your clinic, to get their initial consultation, we give them the option to give you a call.

Then we have to define the button type. For us, it's going to say, "Call Holly" and we're just going to put the phone number that is going to be used when they press that button.

As soon as you're done with that, you've completed your lead generation form, you can save it to use it in the future, finish and you're done.

So, they're going to see the ad. As soon as they click on "Book Now" it's going to jump onto the lead form, and they're going to fill in their details.

Most of the time the details fill in automatically, so they won't even have to fill in anything. They press "Submit." As soon as they press Submit, they get to the "Thank You" page and they get to call your business immediately.

Usually I would recommend using the name of one of your CAs or yourself, whoever's going to answer the phone. It's quite powerful to use someone's name instead of "Call Clinic."

Make it as personal as possible. Human to human. Keep it simple. Just so they know there's a human involved in this process. Because they're on Facebook, it's digital, they've applied, they've shared, there's a barrier, but there's a human on the other side of this thing and for us it's Holly. Holly picks up the phone.

Finally, Facebook is going to review your ad and your copy to ensure it conforms to the rules of Facebook.

In order to conform to the rules of Facebook, you cannot call out on someone's pain, for example. So, in the copy, you cannot say, "Are you having back pain?" Facebook will cap that campaign. It won't even let it through. It's an automatic algorithm.

However, there are usually ways you can work around it. For example, "More and more people in Windsor are suffering with back pain." You're not calling out that specific person, but you're making reference to them. So, you can be clever and play around with the copy for you to get past those rules.

Facebook wants to protect its users. You don't want to be aggressive, you just want to focus on the positive side of things, or just be clever with your wording and shape things in your copy so you call out the pain without calling out the person.

So, that is Facebook Ads Manager. It's as simple as one, two, three. Campaign, Ad set, and the Ad.

STEP #6: LEVERAGE YOUR EXISTING CLIENTS

In this chapter, we're going to look at how to sweat the assets within your four walls and leverage existing clients.

- Referrals

- Reactivation

- Testimonials

The Power of Referrals

So, what is consistently regarded as the most valuable source of new customer in just about any business?

Everyone wants referrals. Everyone's like, "Referrals, referrals, referrals."

However, one of my pet hates… is when I see someone bragging about them having an "only referral" based practice.

Of course, we want lots of referrals, but it's an "and" conversation. Why not have a ton of referrals and Facebook clients. Why not have a ton of referrals and screening clients.

Everything is an "and" conversation. No one is saying that referrals are not amazing, they are amazing.

So, here's the problem. Client referrals are, without doubt, one of the most effective ways to grow any business.

In fact, honestly, if we really could choose just one source of clients and magically have as many as you can handle… you would choose referrals all day long.

Mostly because, it costs about 8 - 10 times more to acquire a new customer as opposed to referrals or reactivation clients.

Having worked with hundreds of chiropractors, I can honestly say that the busiest chiropractors get a very regular stream of referrals. Most of the time when we look at the numbers of one of my associates that's struggling, they will normally at some point lay blame on the fact that they're not getting enough new clients.

Client referrals are, without doubt, one of the most effective ways to grow any business.

When you break down the statistics, on average, every chiropractor in our company gets at least five new clients a week. Across a year, that's our average. Then you look at a few of them and for whatever reason, their average is literally double.

So, everyone else is averaging five and there'll be one or two outliers that have doubled.

When you break down the statistics, we are generating the same number of new clients for them. They're getting the same number of new clients from Facebook, they're getting the same number of new clients from talks, you name it. The big difference is that they will turn a client into another client. So, that's almost double.

It's definitely got something to do with abundance. Even the Bible says that to him that has, more shall be given.

The biggest thing that I can say is that necessity drives away opportunity. When you need new clients, there's no new clients. When you're very busy and don't "need" new patients, that's normally when there queuing up to see you.

What I see with my top docs is they turn a client into another client.

So, there is no doubt that the most experienced chiropractors will always have more new clients than everyone else because they're really good at generating internal referrals.

I can't tell you where I've got this figure from but it's a nice solid number to aim for and that is having about 50% of your clients coming from internal referrals is a great goal. My busiest docs are around there. The weaker docs are nowhere near there. It's just what we see.

And it's got nothing to do with their sources. A lot of people will say, "Yes, but if I'm generating so many new clients online, then obviously my ratio is going to be down." That's just not what we see. It's because what I see with my top docs is they turn a client into another client.

Another point to mention now is the often unmeasured effect that a referral has on your ROI statistics. So, with your return on investment we are working out the lifetime value of a client without considering that, let's say, every three of ten clients refer you someone. How do you measure that? It can be a little difficult.

But it's just worth considering that when you're working out what you can spend on marketing based on your lifetime value, it's actually higher than that.

The Problems with Referrals

But here's a problem with internal referrals. The problem with internal referrals is by most people's definition of internal referral, it is passive, meaning that there's not much you can do to generate an internal referral.

Let's assume that you are doing a great job. I am happy to assume that anyone reading this book is a great practitioner, that you're a great student of your craft, you're great at creating an environment for your clients.

But the problem with referrals is that, generally speaking, they're perceived as passive, meaning besides really creating a great environment and really doing great at giving them a great experience, there isn't much else you can do to create a steady flow.

Assuming you're creating that great experience, you've got to just sit and wait, right?

While a large portion of referrals may happen passively, you will without doubt speed up that process and double the numbers by having a distinct plan.

You may be thinking, "What are you talking about? How do I generate this plan?"

Well, shortly, I'm going to teach you exactly how we generated over 3,000 referrals last year.

I promise you now if I just sat back and wait for referrals, it wouldn't be in the thousands. But we generated over 3,000 referrals last year because we had a distinct plan.

But let's talk about some traditional methods first.

Business Cards and Vouchers

The first thing I want to talk about is handing out vouchers and business cards. And I know you're thinking, "Ryan, I don't need to read a book to know to hand out vouchers and business cards. Are you kidding me?"

But let me ask you this. Are you handing out ten a day? Are handing out ten a week? Not so old school is it? That's the thing, most of the time our bankers are right under our nose.

If you hand out ten a week, that's 500 a year. That's why I like to measure how many vouchers are being handed out at the front desk, because when they say, "I'm handing them out," I hate to take their word for it.

Now I know how many vouchers are at the front desk. So, we can count them, we count how many we are delivering to the clinics.

So, if every single person in your clinic got a referral voucher or a special discount voucher for a loved one, you would get more referrals.

But 10 per week, 500 a year, people are going to take action of that. I'm telling you it's going to be a huge return on investment. I mean if you can hand out 10 per day, it's amazing but even just 10 per week.

So, my recommendation is that while you can have a special coupon at the front desk, don't have a discount or special offer on the business card. They are separate things.

Look, every client that gets offered a special, you want them to feel just that, you want them to feel special.

So, the best results I've seen with this stuff, including in other businesses I run, is when you take out a card and you meet somebody, say, "Listen, I want you to come in. I'm going to give you a card."

You take it out and you write something on it. They don't know what you're writing. Say, "Listen, I've just written a discount on there, so make sure you show them this," and you sign your name.

You make a big deal of it. Say, "When you come to the front desk, please make sure you show them this. I've signed my name, I'm the owner, so with this, they'll give you a free appointment. All you have to do is pay for x-rays."

You can make the offer whatever you decide. I recommend a free appointment.

You probably had a discussion about what's going on, that's what I'd recommend. But you want to do that specific action that makes them feel special.

You want to go, "Listen, I tell you what. I'm going to give you a card. When you come through, just make sure you show them this card because I've written you'll get a special discount with this at the front desk. That's yours. Come whenever you can."

Now do you think that'll make a better impression than just handing them a card and saying, "Come in to see me"? A much bigger impression.

You want to make it look like it's just for them. So physically write on it, sign your name on it and then give it to them.

And also tell them what to do, "Phone, go to this clinic, walk in, go to the website," whatever, tell them what to do.

There's an old saying, "Tell them what you're going to tell them, tell them and then tell them what you told them."

So, you can't tell them enough times what to do.

Ninja Move

But I want to just tell you about a little ninja move. Handing out business cards is just a basic thing that you should be doing and it's just bad business practice not to do it.

However, I prefer not giving a business card. An I know I'm going to contradict myself here.

The reason I say that is you should have the business cards with you, but this works even better. I generate more referrals in my business than any of my chiropractors, because, if I start a conversation, I'll tell them I'm a chiropractor.

When you tell someone you're a chiropractor, what do they say to you? "Oh, my back. Oh, I've got something. You need to check it." I will go straight into what I am about to teach you and literally 9 times out of 10 it works a treat.

So, I'll have a conversation with them and I'll say, "You should really come into the clinic. I'll tell you what I'll do. Why don't you come in for a free assessment? If you just give me your name and number, I'll get the team to phone you and we'll get you in right away. I'll get them to phone you right away and we'll get you in for free. All you'll do is pay for x-rays if we need them. How does that sound?"

I literally take their number. Just as an example, recently we were heading to San Diego to a marketing conference. We were in the taxi to the airport. I'm pretty sure I paid for my marketing conference in the taxi drive because of exactly what happened.

I said, "I'm a chiropractor," and he said, "Oh, I've got back pain." So, I said that exact script.

I asked him a few more question and then went down to exactly this. I had my team called him within minutes. It makes a big impact when they get called straight away.

This has never not worked for me. And I do mean never! Never, ever, ever has someone not come in for an appointment when I've done this.

So, there's very little barrier to entry for this and you're leveraging the law of reciprocation.

That's just a little thing that I do every single week. Every single week. My team has seen me do it. They most of the time want to cringe and crawl under a mat when I'm doing it because a lot of chiropractors are embarrassed to promote themselves but I do it religiously.

Increasing Chance of Referrals Passively

Now let's look at how to passively increase your chances of generating referrals. I've said many times in this book that it's not about the content, it's about the context.

So, businesses frequently give very little attention to creating an environment that encourages referrals.

Take every opportunity you can to pre-frame or demonstrate that people refer in this clinic.

Businesses frequently give very little attention to creating an environment that encourages referrals.

In every one of our clinics, we have big display boards up.

So, every single time someone comes in, they see, "A Warm Welcome to Our New Clients." They are all listed out.

Then there's, "A Big Thank You for Your Referrals." You can see all the many people referring listed there.

So, what am I doing here? I'm creating the environment of the busy restaurant and I've letting people know that people refer here.

Now these look a bit amateurish, on purpose. They look a bit all over the shop and that's exactly how they are supposed to look.

I also mention referrals and new clients in the newsletter. It's the same thing. I want them to open that newsletter and see, "Thank You for Your Referrals" and I want them to see, "Welcome to new clients." It's all social proof.

So, does this stuff really make a difference? I'll tell you what. I refuse to find out if it doesn't.

If you said to me that I have to get rid of those boards and I can't ever do that stuff, I would freak out because I don't want to split test this. I wouldn't be prepared to do that.

This stuff works, I'm telling you. Some of the busiest businesses on the planet do it.

Reactivating Old Customers

The biggest misconception that we have as business owners is that if customers or patients aren't returning anymore, it must mean they are dissatisfied.

That leads us to take no action about them but it is costing us a fortune.

So, let's start by considering why clients don't come back and then we'll go on to look at what we can do about it.

Why Clients Don't Come Back

What is the number one reason that clients don't come back after they stopped using your service? It's because they are embarrassed.

I first heard that from one of my business mentors, it was statistically proven when they did studies with people who'd stopped going to use a service.

They asked them, "Why are you not coming in anymore?" Everyone expected to hear that they were dissatisfied with the service.

But the number one reason they don't come back is because they're embarrassed.

Think about it. Have you ever missed an appointment before? Let's say with a hairdresser. Then you see your hairdresser in the supermarket and you run a mile to avoid them. "I'm so embarrassed that I missed an appointment. They must be so pissed off with me. I didn't even phone to cancel. I'm making a bee-line in the opposite direction so I can avoid the situation all together", that's how embarrassment affects the relationship.

> What is THE NUMBER 1 reason clients don't come back after they have "stopped" using the service...
>
> ## They are simply embarassed...
>
> Therefore when you send them a regular communications clearly letting them know you are not "upset" with them, you will automatically get more people coming back!!!

That's exactly how all your clients feel by the way when they see you walking down the street and they haven't come to see you for three months. They are embarrassed.

They're not upset with you. They're just scared that you're cross with them.

That's all they are. They are simply embarrassed.

Therefore, when you send them regular communications clearly letting them know that you're not upset, then you'll automatically get people to come back.

So, let's look at an example campaign that we used to get a whole bunch of "lost" clients to come back.

Example Reactivation Campaign

We decided to include in our campaign males and females who have at least one adjustment.

I don't want to send to anyone who has come to a Report of Findings and didn't move forward. It's not that I don't try to reactivate this group. We do other campaigns for them.

By the way, from many years of working with probably more associates than anyone on the planet, I will tell you this. On average, 40 percent of most chiropractors' clients are leaving after Report of Findings.

That's 40 percent of all the clients you generate are leaving without having an adjustment. They are not coming back for day three.

That's just what I find after years of working with hundreds of people. Whether you realize it or not, that's probably what's happening.

We need to do something about that, but for this campaign, I only want to talk to people who have at least had an adjustment.

Another requirement I had was that they were older than 20. There's no point in sending it to people younger than that, it's just not our primary demographic. I don't even send emails to anyone under 20.

On average, 40 percent of most chiropractors' clients are leaving after Report of Findings.

Then we have to decide what classifies them as inactive, how long they haven't been in for. This is up to you. But we do 12 weeks and we've done eight weeks before.

It doesn't really matter. It's just having a clear idea.

So, we go back through our lists to find people that meet those criteria and haven't been in for at least 12 weeks.

If they've been in in the last 12-week period, then we classify them as active.

Then we have to decide how far back in our records we go. We've gone back 18 months for our Christmas campaign and, for our Easter campaign, we've gone back two years. You can go back to when you started or first opened if you like. It is up to you, just test a few variations on each campaign.

Here's an additional ninja move by the way. I always like to know how big the list is of people that have spent, say, over $500 or over $1,000.

I will tell you that if you do this you will outperform all your competitors.

If your loyal clients have been with you for four years but they have not been in for three months, I want to know that. Because, if they've had 30 adjustments with me over years, I would happily invest a little bit more to speak to them.

This is where most people go wrong is they'll say, "There's no way that I'm sending a whole bunch of letters." A lot of the experts are going to tell you that you need to send three letters or physical mail pieces. Statistically that gives better results.

What I do is I take the most valuable list, and then I decide, instead of sending the whole say 5,000 of them 3 letters, I'm going to send the top spenders a physical letter or 3. And I will also mix up the media and also potentially add a phone call and a few text messages, but just to that smaller higher spend list.

Now you're getting a lot more bang for your buck because those are hyper responsive buyers from the past. You can afford to do it a bit more to try reactivate them. This also helps with a capacity issue we all have in out practices. So intead of trying to make 5000 phone calls, maybe the shortend more targeted list is just 500. I find that this far more achievable to put in front of your team and still have great results.

Then if you segment further to your top 1%-10% spenders you may decide to add a personal video in email to just them. Again its just more achievable and makes a massive difference to the response rate.

Getting and Using Powerful Testimonials

I want to talk about demonstrating social proof via testimonials. It's a slightly different topic but remember it's not about the content, it's about the context.

So, when you're looking at asking someone for a testimonial, I want you to consider the following facts about testimonials. What someone else says about your product or service is at least a thousand times more powerful than what you say about it.

The ironic thing is that most chiropractors are terrible at asking for testimonials. We feel weird about it.

> **If someone fills out a testimonial form for your business, their lifetime value goes up.**

I want to tell you this one statistic that might change your mind. It doesn't matter what business you're in, this simple statistic shows that if someone fills out a testimonial form, there lifetime value goes up. Just the act of writing the testimonial has a correlation with them staying longer.

We don't know exactly why, but my guess is that if someone writes a positive testimonial... which 99% of people will, if they agree to write a testimonial in the first place ... then it's a lot harder for them to justify the decision of not coming to you anymore.

If they are going to go along the lines and say things like, "They changed my life. I had life changing results. I can sleep better, I can have a better relationship with my family. 20 years of this and nobody was able to help me," now they have subconsciously committed way, way, way more to staying under your care or with your service.

I know this sounds obvious but here are some of the subtle but very important things that people frequently miss when considering a testimonial.

So, this is just business 101. I didn't learn this from chiropractic. But the fact of the matter is that just getting someone to fill out a testimonial form increases your retention with them.

Now, the next thing I want you to consider. This is the basic formula for a testimonial. It's Before, After, After (now). "Before I came to see Dr. Neil, I was like this. After I saw Dr. Neil, that was gone. Now, I play with my kids all the time and it's amazing."

The reality of it is, most of the time when you're asking for testimonials, you're simply just saying to someone, "Please tell us about your positive experience at the clinic."

So, if you had the opportunity to ask questions in a video testimonial, this is what you want to be thinking, Before, After, After.

Testimonial Secrets

- Before, After, After (now)
- Bringing up "scepticism" within the testimonial
- Many people are afraid that
- Demonstarting length of time in practice
- Talking about a friend referring them
- Unexpected benefits
- Talking about the benefits of coming long term

"Before I came to Ryan, my business was in a lot of trouble. After I did the New Patient Avalanche program, I generated, just on lifetime value, more than $30,000 of business in the six weeks. Now, I'm a lot stronger business person and I know how to market."

The next thing about it, if you've got the opportunity to ask someone questions, it's actually really cool if they bring up some type of scepticism in the testimonial. Although a lot of people are scared to have that in the testimonial.

It doesn't always happen, but I love it when they say, "I was very sceptical about coming to see a chiropractor, because I was really nervous that it was going to hurt. But when I came…"

Because here's the thing, whatever they say in that sceptical part, most of your clients are thinking anyway. So, don't be afraid to bring that up. It's a way to handle that objection through a cleverly placed testimonial.

Say, "Tell us a little more about why you didn't see a chiropractor for so long?" And they'll say, "I was scared. I was nervous. I thought I was going to have to come forever, blah, blah, blah."

Also, take every opportunity you can to demonstrate a certain way that you want your customers to behave in your office.

For example, I love demonstrating length of time in testimonials. I will always try and bring this up if I can.

One of the things you want to be bringing up is you want them to be saying, "I've been seeing Dr. Max for four years and before I came..."

You want them saying those things because subconsciously what someone's thinking is, "Gee wiz, they've been coming for four years. This must be good."

However, I don't normally like having number of appointments in there. I've worked in clinics before where we used to have the 20 club, the 30 club, the 40 club, the 100 club, based on amount of adjustments. It just doesn't really feel that great for me, only because it's too much for a client to handle before they understand the context of what we do. It's too soon.

You need something called "gradience." How do you cook a frog? You cook a frog slowly. If you throw a frog in hot water, it jumps out. If you put a frog in cold water and you boil the water slowly, it stays.

Now I've not tried that of course but the theory is that, to cook a frog, you put them in cold water and then you boil the water slowly.

That's what you want to be thinking with your marketing. So, when someone comes into your clinic, you might not want to say, "I'm going to see you 100 times over your lifetime." You may well see them that many times, but if you told them that from day one, it's just too much for them to handle.

So, demonstrating length of time in a testimonial is fantastically powerful.

Let's demonstrate a referral. "Who were you referred by?" "I was referred by so and so." "What did so and so say to make you want to come in?"

These are all things that you can steer the conversation that way.

I'm just giving you this background information because, if you do get the opportunity, it will come up with you subconsciously. Also, if you see this stuff in testimonials, you'll be able to choose the really good ones.

Sometimes you've got a lot of testimonials and you've got to choose a few but now that you know this information, you'll be like, "Oh my word, that one, she actually brought scepticism up there. She told us how long she's been coming. She told us she was referred by a friend."

Another point is unexpected benefits that they had, they never expected to have.

Another one is the benefits of coming long term. The key is that it needs to be conversational and real and subtle. I hope that helps with testimonials. It really would be an injustice for me not to help you understand that concept.

Probably the number one point that you really need to understand is just the concept that simply by filling out a testimonial form, people will stay with your business longer.

The best time to ask for a testimonial is the point of highest pleasure. When they walk out of the room and they say to the front desk, "Oh my word, Dr. Lee is a miracle worker. I feel so good," that is when your front desk needs to go, "Would you mind just sharing that with us on this form?" So, you've got to train your front desk.

STEP #7: PROFIT FROM HOLIDAY CAMPAIGNS

Nothing has created a massive influx of new clients more cheaply and faster for us than leveraging the power of event-based marketing.

I'm going to talk here about how we leverage holidays such as Easter, Christmas, Halloween and Valentine's Day to leverage referrals.

I've put this chapter last because I've now taught you all the elements you need to know for a successful holiday campaign. There's a Facebook element to get new clients and there's a reactivation element by emails and mixed media.

So, this is bringing it all together except for one part I haven't taught you, which is why holidays?

It's all leveraged around events where there is already so much hype in the marketplace, meaning everyone does it.

When do you start seeing Easter Eggs in the shopping markets? Weeks if not months before Easter. Last year, I saw Christmas decorations in October. Because it's heading up to Christmas, nobody even blinks an eye.

So, there's a great justification to market something. It comes across less salesy because everybody is doing it. So, you can say, "Hey, we've got a Christmas special" and it's got a different feel.

The beautiful thing about event-based marketing it's got a start date and an end date, meaning you leverage something powerful in marketing called scarcity to massively increase your response rate.

Easter now runs an entire month, even though it used to just run on the weekend. Halloween is one day but it's Halloween month. It's the month of love for Valentine's. So, you've got an opportunity to leverage that for much longer. It's a very legitimate reason to offer a special.

This is why I truly believe you don't need a marketing calendar besides noting when you have screenings and holiday events.

There's a never-ending list of holidays to market. We have spoken about your Seinfeld emails and when we send these, we almost always leverage it around a national holiday.

I subscribe to a calendar that every day, just tells me today's national holidays.

Just to give you an example, look at February alone:

- February 1 is ... Serpent Day
- February 2 is ... Purification Day
- February 3 is ... Cordova Ice Worm Day
- February 4 is ... Create A Vacuum Day
- February 5 is ... Disaster Day
- February 6 is ... Lame Duck Day
- February 7 is ... Charles Dickens Day
- February 8 is ... Kite Flying Day
- February 9 is ... Toothache Day
- February 10 is ... Umbrella Day
- February 11 is ... White Tee-Shirt Day and Don't Cry Over Spilled Milk Day
- February 12 is ... National Plum Pudding Day
- February 13 is ... Get A Different Name Day
- February 14 is ... Ferris Wheel Day and National Heart to Heart Day
- February 15 is ... National Gum Drop Day
- February 16 is ... Do A Grouch a Favor Day
- February 17 is ... Champion Crab Races Day
- February 18 is ... National Battery Day
- February 19 is ... National Chocolate Mint Day
- February 20 is ... Hoodie Hoo Day
- February 21 is ... Card Reading Day

- February 22 is … Be Humble Day

- February 23 is … International Dog Biscuit Appreciation Day

- February 24 is … National Tortilla Chip Day

- February 25 is … Pistol Patent Day

- February 26 is … National Pistachio Day

- February 27 is … International Polar Bear Day

- February 28 is … Public Sleeping Day

- February 29 is … National Surf and Turf Day

February 5th is Disaster Day. That's awesome to market to. Imagine your subject line, "Are you having a disaster day? Did you know today is disaster day and we really want to make sure that isn't happening in your life. So, on national disaster day, we have come to the rescue."

Umbrella Day, "We've got you covered, it's umbrella day." It just goes on and on and on. Just Google, national holiday calendar's and you will find it.

The reason I've told you that, was because, especially for your Seinfeld emails, there's always an excuse to send the email. You can never not find a holiday to market to. But, I'll give you the big six holidays that we do in a moment.

However, I just want a quick disclaimer here. When it comes to local level marketing, the stuff I'm teaching you now, is not sexy.

So, I want you to understand that most local business campaigns don't work, not because of the validity of the campaign, because I clearly showed you that it does work. But rather because of poor planning, poor follow through and inadequate support.

This is very, very important. I promise you it works but it takes planning and it takes follow through and it takes support of your team. I'm going to teach you how to do that now.

Dan Kennedy says, "Commitment is way more important than creativity."

We do the same five campaigns every year and I've got the whole thing filed, documented and systemized.

One of the biggest lessons for us last year was that we had this slogan, "We're going to train our way to success." So, I really want you to think about this whenever you do an event or event-based marketing.

You will get double and triple the results if you simply understand that by planning and executing correctly your results will be exponentially better. You've got to train your way to success.

- It's not the team's fault that they're not doing it.

- It's not the team's fault that they're not handing out the vouchers.

- It's not the team's fault that they're not using the script for every single person

It's our fault, it's my fault. You the business owner, you are in charge of your life. I'm just really passionate about this, that all business owners take 100% responsibility for their life and business.

It changes the way you feel about your business, when you understand that you're in 100% control of your business, it's your destiny.

If you take 100% responsibility for everything that happens, you will think and act differently.

It changes the way you feel about your business, when you understand that you're in 100% control.

It's not the most pleasant thing in the world, because, here's the thing, as I was once taught, your business is the direct reflection of you. Your business is just a mirror and that is a hard thing to hear because guess what? When things are going well, it feels great. But, when things are not going well, guess who you need to have a long hard chat with in the mirror. Me , myself and I!

So, we take the planning for these campaigns very seriously.

Planning for our Christmas campaign, for example, each meeting is 90 minutes and, if I had to guess, I'd say actual hours sitting working on it was anywhere from 12- 24 hours when we ran it for the first time ever. Now that we have it down, the planning and implementation is a lot quicker, but even then, you've got to dedicate at least a 90-minute meeting to planning for this sort of thing. You probably think this sounds like a lot of work. And it is.

But I just want to share this. I've had the privilege of having many meals with the owners of Success Resources, Veronica and Richard Tan. These are the guys that promote some of the biggest speakers in the world like Tony Robbins and Robert Kiyosaki. They are the biggest event company on the planet. They run at least 500 events a year.

Richard's a Singaporean chap who's a very funny, very cool guy. He's worked very closely with all these people. You can link a lot of Tony Robbins' success and a lot of the Rich Dad empire's success to Richard Tan.

I was sitting down at dinner and I said to Richard, "What are you up to, what projects?" And what he said next I was very impressed with, he said, "I'm busy building a hotel in Singapore."

I said, "Wow Richard, that is unbelievable, that must be so much hard work." And he said these words, "Ryan big project, little project, same work."

It really made an impact on me. I'll never forget it. All I said back to him was, "That's so true."

Richard Tan has the same amount of time as you and I, he's building a hotel with his time, what are we doing with ours.

So, you might as well do this properly when you do it. You're going to have to spend 90 minutes to do it at all, so you might as well spend three to six hours and do it really, really well.

Three Elements to a Holiday Campaign

There are three elements that you must have in every holiday campaign – new clients, reactivations and referrals.

So, in our 'New Year, New You' Christmas offer, we generated 550 new clients from internal referrals. That's close to 70 new clients, per clinic, over about a six-week period.

We also generated 550 from internal referrals and 183 new leads.

Now, you might ask are these people that were going to come in anyway? My most accurate guess is there's no way that we would've got as many leads and referrals if we didn't wrap it around a campaign.

So, you've got these three major elements which you should have in every holiday campaign:

The 3 "Thou Shalt's" of a Successful Holiday Campaign

1. Thou Shalt have: a Referral Element and incentive
2. Thou Shalt have: a Reactivation Element (Mixed media)
3. Thou Shalt have: a New Patient Element (mostly Facebook)

You've got four or five events that you repeat every year that include those three elements.

This is exactly what we do, every single campaign, we go, "Right, it's Valentine's Day. What are we going to do for our referral campaign? What are we going to do for our reactivation elements? What are we going to do for the new patient element?"

We've already covered the steps that you need to follow for most of those – email marketing, Facebook, retargeting, postcards, text messages.

Remember, don't just plan when your going to send emails. Also think a few steps further. When are we going to send them a text and who are you going to send a text to? Who are you going to send the letter to? Maybe it's only your top 2%, but decide who you are going to send the letter to.

I know I sound like a broken record for this but go the extra mile in the planning to work up what your mixed media is.

Every time we take time to plan it, we do better. So, first element, a referral element. Next element, a reactivation element and the last element is a new patient element.

You can see why I did this last, because now you're going to bring it together. I know what's going to happen. There is so much to do, you're going to get overwhelmed. So, I've broken down this simply.

If all you did was get disciplined to do these five campaigns each year and you did these three elements in each campaign and then you ticked away with your; Facebook talks, corporate talks, screenings and your referral stuff, you would have a record year, because you are bringing all those elements into it.

The Big Six Holiday Campaigns

So, here's the big six that we market every year. This is your marketing calendar on one page.

- Christmas/New Year – "New Year, New You" (Mid December to 31 January)

- Valentine's Day (5 February to 28 February)

- Easter campaign

- Summer campaign

- Back to School

- Halloween

We normally do a corporate month too, somewhere around summer, where we do a fishbowl campaign.

Often people freak out and say, "Oh, but it feels like there's just one after the next."

Please remember that not all the exact patients were there the week you did the Christmas campaign, that are there for the Easter campaign. So it's new for them all the time.

The other thing is, we've worked out that if you have a two to three-week break between each campaign, that's normally enough time for everyone to forget about it and feel refreshed but even if you only chose to do 3 per year instead of 6, if will be a huge boost for the practice.

In fact, often it takes two to three weeks to plan these things on our scale.

There are only six campaigns. If you did each campaign for a month, that's six months of the year, so you should normally have a bigger break, but some of them are a little bit closer together.

12 Steps to a Successful Holiday Campaign

This is kind of like a checklist we use to keep us on track each campaign.

There must always be one or one in the pipeline. In our marketing meeting, one of our agenda points that we bring up purposely every week, is upcoming events. We're either in one or we're planning one. There must always be one or one in the pipeline.

12 Steps to a Successful Holiday Campaign

1. There must "always" be one, or one in the pipeline
2. There must be calculated, well thought out planning
3. There must be an "offer" ie 50% off, Free, 80% off, buy one get one free
4. There must be a start date and an end date
5. There must be a team incentive
6. There must be a client "incentive" (regulation dependent)
7. There must be "props" (vouchers, chocolates)
8. There must be fanfare (decoration, dress up)
9. There must be mixed media (email, text, phone, print)
10. There must be a ONE PERSON responsible
11. There must be measurement AND reporting (public)
12. There must be a debrief meeting

There must be calculated well thought out planning.

There must be an offer. Don't wimp out on this. It's a direct response marketing rule. There must always be an offer.

There must be a start date and an end date. Most of the success in these campaigns has really got to do with the end date.

Every single bit of communication with the client is, "It's buy one get one free as long as you book before..." "You can get a free massage if you refer someone as long as you book them in before...". So, there must always be a start date and an end date.

There must always be a team incentive. There must be a client incentive, regulation dependent.

There must be props – vouchers, Easter eggs, golden ticket chocolates. There must fanfare, meaning, decorations, dress ups.

There must be mixed media. So, when you think about your reactivation, always mixed media.

There must be one person responsible. Now, normally when I say this, the question that comes up is, "Mary and Peter are going to share the responsibility of the Christmas campaign." Not allowed.

That is what we like to call, in business, a two headed monster. If more than one person's responsible, nobody's responsible.

That does not mean that one person has to do everything, but one person in your team has to take full responsibility.

I'm going to make a bit of a soft rule that none of the doctors are allowed to be that person. It should be someone on your team.

But one person is responsible. That means calling the meetings, making sure everything's printed, making sure communication has gone out, making sure you're having your product meetings, etc.

There must be measurement and reporting. Normally, the person that's responsible doesn't have to do all the measurements and reporting, but they could delegate and go, "I do need some help from you, Neil or Andrew or whoever to please give me this stat on a weekly basis."

There must always be a debrief meeting after the event. Normally a debrief meeting runs like this: "What happened? Results, what worked, what didn't work," or, "What happened, what worked and what can we do better next time?"

That by the way, is basically every single debrief you'll ever do in your business.

Three Secrets of a Referral Campaign

In this segment, mostly I'm going to focus on referrals because I have already covered the other two elements in more detail.

I just really want to hit this home, so you can get the most out of this. This is your lowest hanging fruit. We did 70 in our last campaign, you can easily generate 20 to 50.

The 3 Secrets that easily generate 20–50 referrals each campaign

- Secret #1 – ask CORRECTLY...
- Secret #2 – Must have BOTH a client AND TEAM incentive!
- Secret #3 – Measure, Measure, Measure!

Now, don't be distracted by those numbers because if you did this and generate 10, it's worth the three hours that you put into plan it.

There are three secrets to creating a successful referral campaign within the whole event.

This will help make sure that you can get double the numbers that you're currently getting but it takes getting help from your team to do this.

- First, you've got to ask correctly.

- Next, you must have both a client incentive and team incentive.

- And the last element is, you must measure, measure, measure.

Secret #1: Ask Correctly

First secret, ask correctly. If I had a penny for every single time I'd heard a coach, or somebody say that the way you get referrals is just ask, I would be a very wealthy man.

We've all heard people say that, but what irritates me about that is it's a lot easier said than done. It's actually quite awkward to ask for a referral, it's actually quite a challenging thing.

So, I'm going to break it down to three steps.

I was once taught this… if you turn all your statements into questions, you will go very far in life.

With that in mind, this is the basic script for asking for a referral.

First, you're going to say this to someone, and your team needs to know this, "Have you been told about our said special?"

"Hey John, have the front desk told you about our free Royal Wedding special?"

Basis "Asking: Script

1. Have you been told about "SAID SPECIAL"?
   (Pause for answer)
2. Tell them
3. Who would you like to…?

Now it's important that you stop talking here because then what's going to happen is they'll say, "No, nobody's told me about the special."

Now you have permission.

I've said this a few times in this book, it's really about permission-based marketing, it's really about trying to get permission.

It's the same with Facebook and even on the emails. The reason I've got the button in there is because I want to have permission to call someone. When someone says, "Yes, call us back to book an appointment," it just goes to the thank you page and now I've got permission to call them.

Same thing here, "John has somebody told you about our free Christmas special." They're going to say, no. Now you've got permission to tell them what it is and then you're going to finish with another question, "Who would you like to get booked ... ?" That's the whole script.

This sounds really simple, but I promise you, when we got that script printed and laminated at the front desk in every clinic for one of our campaigns our referrals doubled.

The thing is, you will all look at that now and you'll go, "That's pretty basic," but imagine what would happen if even 50% of your clients get asked that sequence. You would massively increase your internal referrals every month.

So, this is what the full script looks like.

> Hey John, has anyone at the front desk told you about the free Valentine's promotion this month?

Or

> John, are you aware of our Valentine's special we have on this month?

They're going to say, "No" and then you tell them what it is. Now there's one more part.

> We are offering a consultation and x-rays for all your friends and family for free (or discount), which is worth up to $110 per person!! The offer is only valid for appointments booked until the ... . Once they have come in, you will be entitled to have a free massage.

This is one of the specials we did. We had a massage therapy college phone us up, they were trained to do massage, and asked if we can help them out to give their people hours.

It was right at Valentine's and I wasn't sure what I was going to do with these people. It then dawned on me that every single person who refers someone could get a free massage and also the person that got referred.

I was an amazing campaign and it was just a coincidence, it all happened at once.

Then, there's a very important question at the end of the paragraph:

Sound good, yes? (It's important to get a yes)

Whatever offer you give someone, if you say that, "Sounds good, yes?" and then they say yes, statistically, it's been shown if you get five yeses in a row, you can massively increase conversions.

Then you ask:

Who would you like to get booked in before our special ends, your wife, your children, parents? PAUSE ....

"Who can we get booked in?" that's all you ask and here's the key. The big thing that stops people from asking is fear of rejection.

The success of internal referral campaigns has way more to do with the front desk than it does with the chiropractors.

So, I really want to give you this little analogy that really helped me serve at higher level.

When you're offering anything; chiropractic services, coaching, whatever it is, you've really got to come from this energy high intention. You want people to come and see you, you want to convert people, you want people to stop having pain, you want to help them. You sell the best product on the planet so why wouldn't you really want them to come in. But, part of selling successfully is to have this high intention and while at the same time maintaining low attachment to the result. High intention, you want to help people a lot, but low attachment to the results.

It gives you permission to ask as many people as you can about the Christmas special, whatever it is but if no one takes it up, it's okay.

Studies have shown that sometimes people have to hear something seven times before they buy. So, the key point of this whole thing is to make it successful. If you just stood in the room, it will be successful but if you and your front desk do it together, that's when you're going to get your big punch.

I'm honestly a massive believer that the success of internal referral campaigns has way more to do with the front desk than it does with the chiropractors. With my next secret, you'll understand why.

Secret #2: Must Have Both a Client and a Team Incentive

Secret number two – you must have both a client and a team incentive. Let's talk about the client incentive first.

So, what's our client incentive? Client incentive can be a free appointment. We don't ever do this actually for a referral, but I just wanted to mention it. It is an option, and would it make sense financially? You're darn right it would, but I don't do this.

Or you can say 50% off your next appointment or you can say there's a free massage or you simply just send a thank you card.

Now my disclaimer with this is that in some parts of the world sometimes you can't offer an incentive for a referral. But even if you can't incentivize someone to refer, you must always thank them.

One of the things we did was to just put a lotto ticket in their referral thank you card. And here's the thing, there's such a high perceived value for it, but it's just a piece of paper that's worth virtually nothing - $2 or whatever it is. But it's just a cool little thing that we like to do.

Just do whatever feels right for you.

Again, it goes back to a lifetime value. It doesn't really matter what your lifetime value is, but if your lifetime value is $800, $1,000, $2,000 and you don't take the time to say thank you, you will lose out.

By the way I'm not immune to this. There have been times when we were not doing it religiously and it was a real wake up call for me.

The marketplace will always tell you exactly whether you did a good job or bad job.

If you're not serving that marketplace, if somebody gave you a referral and you're not recognising it, think of the laws of Yin and Yang and Karma and all those things, if you don't at least show your appreciation for that, the universe is probably not going to give you much more.

There's an old saying that you cannot have more, until you appreciate what is. So, every single time someone is referred, we send a little card to whoever referred them.

So, if all you got from this chapter is you start doing that, you will get more referrals.

If someone does anything good for you, try to say thank you. When you do something nice for someone else you want a thank you. If that's all you did is send a thank you for the referral, it would be fantastic.

This philosophy also goes for appreciating and surprising new patients. We've recently started sending every single new patient a welcome pack in the post. Its been a fantastic initiative we have introduce and its decreased our no show rate and gives us an opportunity to position ourselves the way we want to before they walk in. There's a little spine keyring in there a welcome letter and they get testimonials and celebrity testimonials and our most recent newsletter that has been strategically chosen as its has a Q&A section in it that specifically deals with the common objections I believe that a lot of new patients may have prior to walking in the door or stopping them from taking up care.

Incentives have doubled our results in certain cases.

I'm telling you this, when you start in this marketing world, you start by thinking that marketing's about getting as many people through the front door as you can. Then you start looking at these things a little differently than just getting them through the front door. You start thinking about how you can effect "how" they show up. How to stack the decks in your favour before they walk in.

A note on team incentives. You can do a lot of great stuff by yourself, but you can achieve anything with a team. So, this is where the magic lies.

Incentives have doubled our results in certain cases. It's the quickest way to get all your team look in the same direction. This is how we do it – little targets.

Numbers are great, but it means more to the chiropractor than it does to the front desk.

When you have multiple little campaigns, you need to get people constantly looking in the same direction.

Let me give you an example. This is why you need to document all your previous years. Last year at Christmas we generated 550 new clients by internal referral. So, this year my goal will be at least that for my team.

Then, if we hit that we have a new little incentive. I've done this many times and we've only really just got the hang of it now. Let's say the goal is that we want to hit 200 a week, 300 a week, whatever. Straight away the energy is up and if you follow the golden rules, you have an incentive and the guys work really hard and now hit 300.

Then, directly after that, what do you think happens to numbers? They tank or drop dramatically.

It shows how powerful it is though, so I want you to watch for the peak and then the falling off the cliff, meaning that the team will work really hard to hit it and once they hit it, they lose energy and numbers will drop dramatically.

This works best if there's a little competition amongst the CAs or the practitioners or multiple clinics. We leverage this big time.

We find that experiential rewards work the best. We don't really give money rewards; the odd one we do.

Experiential rewards are things like spa days, team meals. We've gone to fancy restaurants; we've sent the whole team on spa days. In one case, everyone from the winning practice went to theatre in London, and they had everything paid for. There are so many things you can do.

Then, for our biggest reward we send the whole team to Ibiza if they hit it. Paid for, flights and accommodation. Pretty cool!

Working Out Targets and Incentives

So, how can you justify this stuff? It all comes back down to the basics.

Earlier on, I spoke about the three most important numbers that you have to know:

1. Lifetime value

2. Cost per lead

3. Cost per client

But really, the top two, lifetime value and cost per lead, if you know that, you can work out any campaign.

This is how you work out a target and how you work out an incentive.

Let's say you've worked out your target based on numbers per week, and you work out that if you hit those numbers, the extra revenue in the business is $1,000 per week.

If you do that for four weeks, for instance, that is $4,000 extra in the business that month.

Most people go, if my incentive costs me $500 or $200, then obviously it's worth it to get $4,000 which makes sense but what everyone forgets about is the value that you created in your business on the way to hitting the target.

What about all the weeks where they just miss it? What about all the weeks where it's creeping up?

Let's say increased revenue over four weeks was $400, $300, $250, $800. That's already an extra $1,750. If you add that to the $4,000, that's the total return on investment.

Now, don't worry, don't go to the efforts of working out what it was worth to you in the weeks you weren't hitting it. They say the first part change, is awareness so I just want you to bring that into your consideration.

But, if it drives everything up, it's even more worth it because in the long run you're driving the business up in a big way.

If you subtract the cost of the campaign from that, what you'll work out is your profit. I've banged on about this the whole book, but knowing your numbers is important.

I can tell you that people thought we were crazy when I said we're going to send people to Ibiza. We sent 60 people to Ibiza. Flights, accommodation paid for. That set us back thousands upon thousands of dollars.

It's all relative, because you guys are spending in the same way, just to a different scale. It sounds a lot more, but you've got to understand that your return on investment's already there.

So, how do you prevent this peak and then falling off the cliff? You need to set way more achievable goals that you are. That's probably the opposite of what you expected from me.

In the beginning, let's say you want 250 a week. What a lot of people do is one off, "Hit 350 and then we'll all go to Ibiza."

The problem with that, is that that lends itself very much to the hitting the target and then falling off the cliff.

What I prefer now is way more modest targets, in fact, sometimes I will set targets on numbers we've already hit.

That's the best, when it makes sense, we just set the target on numbers we've hit in the past. But you just do it for longer time periods. I want consistency.

So, let me give you an example. Let's say you're on 250 a week and you want to get to, whatever it is. Instead of saying 350, you might say, "Look chaps, we've hit 300 once or twice, if we just keep it at 300 for three consecutive weeks or three weeks in a quarter, we've hit our target." That's much better.

Or you could say, "For at least four weeks in a given period, we have to hit that number. Or three weeks of that number this quarter."

What we've done for our current one, we actually broke it up into two quarters. So, they have to hit the target three times this quarter and three times in that quarter. But now it's capped. So now they have to hit it in both quarters. Very powerful.

It also prevents low morale when they don't hit the massive targets.

Some of our targets only be set at 5%, 10%. This year, across the board, I think we looked at 15%. So, when you look at 15% in a clinic, it's tiny. Let's say the clinic is on 300, then you're not looking at a massive amount of growth. But they have to hit it consistently it makes a big impact.

So, that's my suggestion for that. I know it happens. I've worked with so many people with this. They'll set the target and then, because you've set a target, your team will hit it and you'll go, "Oh, my word, I set it too low."

That's not the point, you want your team to hit the target. It's not, "Hopefully they don't hit it, so I don't have to pay for the prize."

You want your team to hit the target. So, just make sure it's more achievable for a longer period. That's what my suggestion would be.

That's why it's so important to measure everything so you can use it as a reference point. Now next year I know exactly what our targets are because I've measured and documented this year's and last year's results.

Secret #3: Measure, Measure, Measure

Secret number three: Measure, measure, measure. I've been really big on this the whole book. Whenever you want something to improve in your business, you simply need to measure it.

But Pearson's law takes it further. When performance is measured and reported, the rate of improvement accelerates. It actually says it's exponential. When it's measured and reported on, it increases exponentially.

When I hear a law like that, it becomes a golden rule in my business. So, I want to show you what we do. The stuff I'm teaching now, it's literally our checklist. We will go, "Why am I not getting results? Guys are you measuring?" "Yeah, we're measuring." "Are you reporting?" And that's often where we fall down.

For example, we set up a campaign for our clinics to get Google reviews. There was a prize for the winning clinic.

It's a very cool campaign. You send someone a text and then they click on a link and they go straight to your Google page and then fill it in. So, we had a competition for the team that sent the most links.

It was crazy how many Google views we generated from this. But we weren't getting traction until we measured it and we put it on our Facebook page, every single week, a name and shame.

We sent 750 texts for some people to fill out and we probably got like 200, 300 reviews from that in a short space of time. But the only reason we got those results is because we measured, and we reported.

Another example was our Christmas campaign and I compared my clinics.

Every week, it's like, "Windsor is in the lead. They got 40 referrals. Surbiton, you guys are behind. New Malden, you're catching up second place."

I promise you this, people will do so much to avoid the shame of this that they will perform at high levels to do it.

Tony Robbins says this, "You are the direct reflection of the expectations of your peers."

So, you want to be in that kind of environment. The tighter the context, the higher your performance because ultimately "performance requires pressure"

IN CLOSING

So now that you know how we built a business that helps thousands of people every single week, I think its important to reiterate one more time that what you have just read IS NOT THEORY. These strategies are from the front line of a busy business that managed to achieve what just 1% of all business on the planet are able to achieve. Having said all that, I leave you with one challenge, TEST TEST TEST.

If you go out an boldly implement these strategies there are a couple things I will guarantee you will happen;

1. Mistake's will be made. That's how you learn. Imperfect action beats perfect procrastination any day.

2. More people will be helped.

3. Chiropractic itself will become more abundant by serving more people.

4. You and your family will become more abundant.

And with that I am excited to hear your progress and wish you all the success and abundance in the world.

Contact me directly at info@dcpracticegrowth.com

ABOUT THE AUTHOR

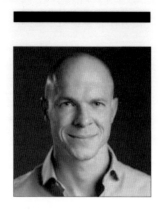

Dr Ryan Rieder is a Chiropractor, husband, father and serial entrepreneur. He grew up and studied Chiropractic in South Africa. After graduating he and his wife Natalie (also a Chiropractor) moved to the United Kingdom where he co-founded Halsa care group. In just 5 years Halsa has grown to 8 offices, several of which are million dollar practices. Halsa now has over 100 team members that serve thousands of patients every single week.

Ryan is also actively involved in helping practices across the globe grow through his tried and tested marketing and business strategies. He is a frequent speaker at Chiropractic events and business growth events across the world, including T Harv Ekers Millionaire Mind Intensive, with him more recently having shared the stage with marketing legend Jay Abraham and Robert Kiyosaki.

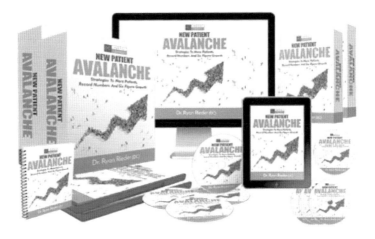

WANT TO FIND OUT MORE?

Log on to dcpracticegrowth.com **now**

 Check out my video show

 Listen and subscribe to my podcast

 Read my latest Growth blog

 Book in for a free strategy call

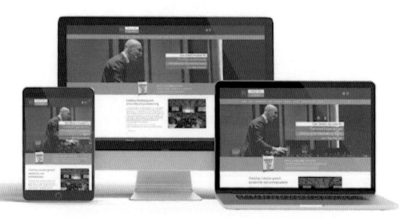

DCPRACTICEGROWTH.COM

CLAIM YOUR AMAZING FREE BONUS

Access your live bonus training of the Facebook platform

- ✓ Learn how to double your new patients using Facebook

- ✓ Learn how to get 60-100 new leads on Facebook in days

- ✓ See the benefits of using Facebook in your practice

- ✓ Spread your message to a whole new audience

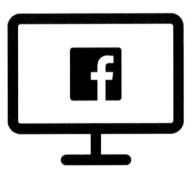

GO TO NPAMARKETINGBOOK.COM TO UNLOCK YOUR FREE BONUS OR EMAIL INFO@DCPRACTICEGROWTH.COM

THE MOST INCREDIBLE FREE GIFT EVER!

GET 3 MONTHS FREE MEMBERSHIP

Learn how to claim your $441 worth of pure, powerful, practice-growing material absolutely FREE! Get our monthly 25+ page "Practice Growth Playbook" sent straight to your door!

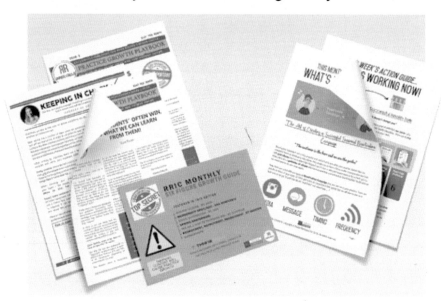

GO TO NPAMARKETINGBOOK.COM/PRACTICE-GROWTH-PLAYBOOK TO UNLOCK YOUR FREE BONUS OR EMAIL INFO@DCPRACTICEGROWTH.COM